# MACHINE DREAMING
# AND CONSCIOUSNESS

# MACHINE DREAMING AND CONSCIOUSNESS

J. F. PAGEL

PHILIP KIRSHTEIN

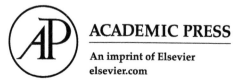

ACADEMIC PRESS

An imprint of Elsevier
elsevier.com

Academic Press is an imprint of Elsevier
125 London Wall, London EC2Y 5AS, United Kingdom
525 B Street, Suite 1800, San Diego, CA 92101-4495, United States
50 Hampshire Street, 5th Floor, Cambridge, MA 02139, United States
The Boulevard, Langford Lane, Kidlington, Oxford OX5 1GB, United Kingdom

**Notices**
Knowledge and best practice in this field are constantly changing. As new research and experience broaden
our understanding, changes in research methods, professional practices, or medical treatment may become
necessary.

Practitioners and researchers must always rely on their own experience and knowledge in evaluating and
using any information, methods, compounds, or experiments described herein. In using such information or
methods they should be mindful of their own safety and the safety of others, including parties for whom they
have a professional responsibility.

To the fullest extent of the law, neither the Publisher nor the authors, contributors, or editors, assume any
liability for any injury and/or damage to persons or property as a matter of products liability, negligence
or otherwise, or from any use or operation of any methods, products, instructions, or ideas contained in the
material herein.

**British Library Cataloguing-in-Publication Data**
A catalogue record for this book is available from the British Library

**Library of Congress Cataloging-in-Publication Data**
A catalog record for this book is available from the Library of Congress

ISBN: 978-0-12-803720-1

For Information on all Academic Press publications visit our
website at https://www.elsevier.com/books-and-journals

# Working together
# to grow libraries in
# developing countries

ELSEVIER   Book Aid International

www.elsevier.com • www.bookaid.org

*Publisher:* Mara Conner
*Acquisition Editor:* April Farr
*Editorial Project Manager:* Timothy Bennett
*Senior Production Project Manager:* Priya Kumaraguruparan
*Designer:* Matthew Limbert

Typeset by MPS Limited, Chennai, India

# DEDICATION

Haskell Wexler
The camera became alive in his hands.

# CONTENTS

# ACKNOWLEDGMENTS

This book was a delight to write, pushing me into fields where my intellect had to be quick, climbing across mixed-rock in a fluid dance, without protection. This project begin in shared presentations with Haskell Wexler on the Science of Story. Much thanks goes again to Kathleen Broyles for her editing and her delightful illustrations that provide insight and lightness in sometimes heavy surf. Richard Moore, the pastoral professor of white whales, pushed the concept of story into the arc of this work. The reader will be appreciative. The calligraphy figure in Chapter 4, Testing for Machine Consciousness, and the cover picture are my own. The cover petroglyph is of a shaman, one of many images on the hunting shrine at Big Arsenic Springs-in what President Obama designated as Rio Grande del Norte National Monument, a place I visit often as a Site Watch monitor for the State of New Mexico. The picture is taken as the sun crests the ridge, just days after the autumn equinox, when the image changes so quickly from moment to moment, that it leaps from the rock, almost alive.

# Machine Dreaming and Consciousness— The Human Perspective

*Sometimes the machine's answer is as hallucinatory and imprecise as any biologically produced dream—a strangely structured, somewhat askew, often hard to remember, altered, and yet often useful alternative view of external experience and reality. (Chapter 9: Interpreting the AI Dream)*

Is it possible that machines might someday possess the potential to dream? For some of us, this potential is disconcerting. For others, it is an imaginative, futuristic reality that possesses hope and unforeseen possibility. In this world, questions of philosophy and metaphysics lie, both at the poorly circumscribed center and the border of neuroscience and computer science. The computer era's discoveries present new problems for philosophers to ponder, new abstractions for artists to illuminate. It has opened doors to new narrative forms, with science fiction bearing some of the burden in the creation of alternate realities. Today's virtual reality borders on Westworld.

This book will take you on an exploration into the world of machine dreams from a scientific perspective. These are areas of mind—definingly human, executive, higher level functions and forms of cognitive operation. It's an attempt to focus on the reality of machine dreams—in terms of what it means to dream, if you are a machine. And what it means to be human if we lose our singular connection to this aspect of our humanity.

Today both neuroscience and computer science are at a nexus, a choke point acting as a bottleneck router, where approaches to developing AI and robotic systems that interact and think like humans, have come up against limitations and borders. Current systems utilizing mathematically logical programming have difficulties interacting in a human common-sense reality functioning without clear logic. In order to be like humans in the same way that humans interact with their own world, it is becoming increasingly apparent that AI and robotic systems require new forms of hardware and software with increased flexibility, and fewer controls. In order to function in our commonsense human world, systems must function less like parametric calculators and more like biological systems. These systems may very well require an equivalent capacity to dream.

In this section, we will address the human perspective and understanding of dreaming (Chapter 1: Dreaming: The Human Perspective), and the convoluted philosophical and scientific path followed in attempting to understand consciousness (Chapter 2: The Mechanics of Human Consciousness). We will explore the known forms of dreaming and consciousness, particularly as alternatively expressed by other animals (Chapter 3: Animal Dreaming—Animal Consciousness). And we will look closely at the tests that we humans have developed in our attempts to define consciousness (Chapter 4: Testing for Machine Consciousness). In the next section, we will delve into the fields of computer science in order to describe the development of operative processing in some ways equivalent to machine dreaming. In the final section, we address the current realities, philosophies, and future possibilities for machine consciousness and dreaming, and explore how any machine capacity to dream is likely to affect those systems, and alter conceptions of our own humanity.

AI consciousness and machine dreaming present dilemmas for many of the philosophers and scientists of today, who have difficulty fully defining either consciousness or dream. We are prone to view the experiences of consciousness and dreaming as special and unique human capacities. Dreams are a primary aspect of the human experience. We now live in a world rushing down the path to creating their artificial equivalents.

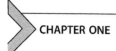

# CHAPTER ONE

# Dreaming: The Human Perspective

*Anthropomorphic: ascribing human forms or attributes to a being or thing not human, esp. to a deity.[1]*

For humans, dreams are a virtually ubiquitous experience. Almost everyone dreams. To each dreamer what a dream is appears to be self evident. Yet being human, conflation and confusion, supposition and presumption abound. What is obviously a dream to one person may not be at all what another is referring to as a dream. Dreams are very different phenomena not only to different dreamers, but also to the various types of scientists, therapists, shamans, and priests who write and study their attributes. If we are to determine whether artificial intelligence (AI) systems have the capacity to experience dream-like cognition, we must first attempt to define what we call dreaming.

There are archeological suggestions that dreams were among the first aspects of cognition addressed by our species. The cave paintings in southern Europe, approximately 35,000 years old, are the oldest artistic artifacts from our species that have been preserved into the present day. These representative renderings were created deep in caves, apparent to their viewers only in the flickering light of lamps used to dispel a total darkness parodying sleep. Like dreams, these are images from the waking Paleolithic world of the painters. Most are of animals, both prey and predators. Displayed in exquisite detail are sexuality, pregnancy, incongruous transitions from animal to human, and violent death. On the floors of the caves are the remnants of lamps, fires, musical instruments, and shrines—evidence, perhaps, of shamanistic ritual (Fig. 1.1).[2] A strong argument can be made that some, at least, of these images were inspired and adapted from dream imagery, from an altered state of consciousness available even then to our species.[3]

The cave paintings suggest that early humans paid attention to their dreams. The paintings also indicate that they understood much about the

*Machine Dreaming and Consciousness.*
DOI: http://dx.doi.org/10.1016/B978-0-12-803720-1.00001-3

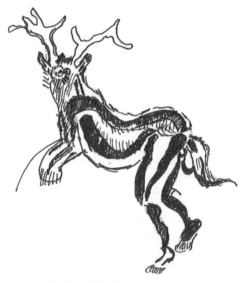

**Figure 1.1** The Sorcerer of Les Trois-Freres.

experience of dreaming. Their dreams occurred primarily during sleep, a state of darkness and perceptual isolation. The images that they created are not detailed pictures of actual experience. They are reflections and representations of experience, their waking world of prey and predator, hunting and escape. The images are outlined, unique, and sometimes moving, standing free of context and scenery. There is much to suggest that at least some of these cave images were derived from dreams. Some have stories, some like those of nightmares, are vicarious, seemingly real experiences of death and dismemberment. The images are emotionally powerful, salient, bizarre, and even sexual. Painted deep in the earth, the focus still today of pilgrimage and ceremony, these images, like dreams, seem spiritual, tied to the phenomena of magic and religion.

Many of these same perspectives of dream persist today. The most powerful determinant of dream content is waking experience—what we now call continuity. Since the Paleolithic, it is waking experience rather than dreams that have changed, so that today we are more likely to dream of the latest ball game or film, than our most recent confrontation with prey or predator.[4] We still make art from our dreams. Artists in creating such dream-based work utilize unique representations and visual patterns taken out of context and scenery, incorporating dream emotions, associations, and images—the alternative and sometimes bizarre understandings we experience in dream—into the creative process.[5]

The earliest decipherable writings are Sumerian codas inscribed on fire-hardened clay over 6000 years ago. Among these is the early inscription of a dream that came to the King of Ladak instructing him in a dream as to how to orient his temple.[6] All of our early religious texts include dreams and nightmares. To the prophet, to the believer, dreams were most often defined as a message from God. Aristotle described a definition as the descriptions of a topic's "essence or essential nature."[7] This was but the first of a series of definitions that were to be used for dream, so that today, there is still not a concrete or set definition for dream to which everyone can agree. Yet when you query any group, there are a series of recurring and set definitions used for dream.[8] Even the oldest of these descriptions are still used and believed by some. And as such, each definition applies and reflects an essence of the state.

## DREAM DEFINITION # 1—MESSAGES FROM GOD

This is one of the oldest and most important definitions ascribed to dreaming, a concept of dreaming that even thousands of years ago created a philosophic conundrum. For surely not every dream, even those of priests and kings, could be a message from the creator. Almost everyone dreams, including such historically marginalized individuals as children, the insane, and women. Some dreams are nightmares, frightening dreams that disrupt sleep, and evidence perhaps, for the existence of personally maligning and terribly negative gods and devils. One of the first questions addressed by the ancient Greek philosophers was the question of true versus false dreams. Homer notes in The Odyssey, "For fleeting dreams have two gates: one is fashioned of horn and one of ivory. Those which pass through the one of sawn ivory are deceptive, bringing tidings which come to nought, but those which issue from the one of polished horn bring true results when a mortal sees them."[9] For many organized religions, primary attributes for God include roles in supplying operative directions for appropriate behavior. Such information is provided by books, teachers/priests, or through personal experiences of contact in prayer, visions, or in dreams. In today's world, particularly among those whose belief systems include the involvement of an active and controlling outside force, dreams may still be interpreted and defined as messages from God. Today the role of the philosopher, the shaman, priest, and the scientist in addressing dreaming remains one of discriminating horn from ivory—delineating that which is true from that which is false.

## DREAM DEFINITION # 2—BIZARRE OR HALLUCINATORY MENTATION

The content of our dreams is often very different from our focused, often logically based experiences of waking consciousness. Developing the approach of psychoanalysis at the start of the 20th century, Sigmund Freud used dreams as a means of access into the process of human psychodynamics. The bizarre and hallucinatory mentation of dreaming was evidence for the existence of unconscious content and systems.[10] Freud proposed that a trained psychoanalyst could utilize such dreams to provide insight into the psychodynamic origin and structure of psychiatric illness.[11]

That psychoanalytic definition of dream (bizarre and hallucinatory mentation derived from the unconscious) is still today one of the most commonly utilized definitions for dreaming. As based on this definition, dream is defined by its content. Such mental activity, called dreaming, can occur during waking as well as during sleep. According to this line of reasoning, dreaming is taking place during sleep only when that reported cognition is bizarre, unusual, and unexpected. The other commonly dreamt, more typical, less bizarre and day-reflective cognition should not really be called dreaming, it is instead sleep-associated thought.[12]

## DREAM DEFINITION # 3—REPORTS OF MENTAL ACTIVITY OCCURRING DURING SLEEP

In the sleep laboratory, dream recall is accessed after an awakening, when the individual is asked to describe, write down, or otherwise report whether a dream has occurred. Dreams are reported from throughout sleep. Recall occurs at highest frequency during sleep onset (stage 1) and during the last REM sleep period of the night (>80% reported recall). Dreams are recalled less often (40% of awakenings) from deep sleep (stage 3) and stage 2.[13] The dreams reported from each stage are different with phenomonologic, eletrophysiologic, and neuroanatomic characteristics associated with each of the sleep stages.[3]

Many variables affect the process of dream recall. Some of the factors affecting dream recall include: time since awakening, type of report, bias and perceived definition for dreaming, sex and attitude of recorder, personality profile of dreamer, and dream intensity and salience.[14] There is no dream recall reported from at least 20% of awakenings, even from the sleep states known to have high recall such as REMS and sleep onset. Because of the multiplicity of variables involved, it is unclear as to whether this lack of recall is a lack of dream remembering or whether it actually reflects episodes of "dreamless" sleep. It is quite possible that some form of dreaming is present when any human is sleeping, but not always recalled or remembered on awakening. Dreaming like thought, as Descartes suggested many years ago, may be a ubiquitous characteristic of an alive and functioning human.[15]

## DREAM DEFINITION # 4—DREAMING IS REM SLEEP

When William Dement discovered rapid eye movement (REM) sleep in the 1960s, he noted that when individuals were awakened from this stage of sleep in which their eyes were moving rapidly back and forth, they most often reported dreaming. His initial speculation suggested that his subjects were dreaming of watching ping-pong or a tennis match.[16] This discovery of REM sleep came at the end of the psychoanalytic era, and with great fan-fair was integrated into psychoanalytic theory. Researchers and theorists adopted the perspective, with almost no proof, that dreaming took place only during REM sleep. REM sleep was interpreted as "smoking gun" evidence that the "primitive" brain stem state of REM sleep was dreaming. REM sleep was evidently equivalent to the psychoanalytic wild child, the mythical "Id," from which bizarre content rose up from primitive aspects of the mind (activation), before being integrated and modulated by higher cortex operating systems.[12] The supposition that REM sleep is dreaming has been incorporated into the most widely accepted theories of neuro-consciousness.[17] Fifty years of neuroscientific and research focus led to remarkable insights into the state. Today, the electrophysiology, neurochemistry, neuroanatomy, and associated physical correlates of REM sleep are among the best described of any CNS state. All physiological activation taking place in the CNS or in the extended body during REM sleep could be viewed as part of dreaming. The dreaming = REM sleep correlate became philosophically and theoretically indispensible. The abundance of data indicating that dreaming occurs without REM sleep and REM sleep without dreaming was ignored and disparaged.

Most neuroscientists became devoted monists. It was seemingly obvious that all aspects of mental functioning (mind) were based on neuroanatomic processing occurring in the brain. The primary empiric evidence supporting this belief was the apparent finding that the biologic brain state of REM sleep was the mind-based state of dreaming. Today, most neuroscientists have been forced to back off, equivocate, and even surrender their belief in the equivalence of REM sleep to dreaming. It is now clear even to long-term supporters that dreaming and REM sleep are doubly dissociable.[18] While REM sleep equals dreaming is losing its cachet, it persists as a definition, an equivalence believed by many, today endlessly reiterated in many popular and college-level texts on sleep.[19] But, empirically it is questionable as to whether there is any special association between REM sleep and dreaming.[20] The primary evidence that the dreams of REM sleep differ from the dreams of the other sleep stages is the finding that the reports of REM sleep dreams are longer and include more words.[21] Nightmares with their negative emotions and frightening content, also typically occur in REMS, except in patients with post-traumatic stress disorder (PTSD). This finding has been used to suggest that REM sleep functions as an emotional processing system.[22] But, emotional processing of negative life events is clearly not restricted to REM sleep. Negative, bizarre, and extremely emotional dreams occur throughout sleep, associated with sleep onset (hypnogogic hallucinations and sleep paralysis), stage 2 (panic attacks), and deep sleep (night terrors and confusional arousals).[3]

## DREAM DEFINITION # 5—A DREAM IS TAKING PLACE WHEN A LUCID DREAMER PUSHES A BUTTON

Lucid dreaming is the capacity to be consciously aware and in volitional control of the dream storyline during the cognitive process of dreaming. Most dreams have a lucid aspect. The dreamer of the dream is almost always a presence in the dream (i.e., all dream stories occur from the perspective of the dreamer's point-of-view). There are some individuals who during episodes of lucidity seem to have the capacity to signal an outside observer that they are dreaming, usually either by pushing a button or by making a series of controlled eye movements. From the perspective of dream science, this is a potentially great technique, perhaps the only technique that can be used to know when a sleeping individual is actually dreaming. But there are problems. Individuals who have the capacity to signal while in lucid dream are rare, so rare, that they may actually be less common than individuals who cannot dream. The most recent major study using this technique (a study well funded, using state-of-the-art technology, and published in a major peer-reviewed journal) was based on the performance of only three subjects. The limited data from that study seems to indicate that when signaling these individuals are in a state that is not clearly either sleep or wake.[23] EEG and scanning data indicate that during signaling the subjects are in a state of awakening that includes visual and motor forms of arousal—what might be better described as a state of controlled sleep off-set.[24] This is not particularly surprising, since REM sleep, the state from within which a majority of lucid dreaming has been reported, is a state that requires for definition the physical occurrence of atonia—the inability to move one's skeletal muscles.[20]

## DREAM DEFINITION # 6—THE FULFILLMENT OF A WISH

Google the topic or peruse the filing system at your local library. Wish fulfillment (dream marriages, dream vacations, dream homes, and dream cars) is the most generally utilized definition for dream. This definition of dream is only very loosely Freudian. Such dreaming is often celebrated in poetry and song as a verb, as in "dreaming the impossible dream."[25] This popular view emphasizes some of the difficulties faced by the field of dream science. As David Foulks, one of the premier scientists of dream has pointed out, "...There is something about dreaming that has always seemed to move people prematurely to forsake the possibility of disciplined empirical analysis."[26] While the other common definitions for dreaming are all based at least in part on suppositions rather than facts, this definition is the one that is most clearly based on a nonempiric logic in which dream is the essence of belief.

## THE PROBLEMS OF DEFINITION

The problem of confused and even contradictory definitions has led to significant problems for researchers and investigators in the fields of dream study. What a dream is to a sleep scientist is not at all what a dream is to the field of psychoanalysis. For the sleep physician dreams occur only in sleep. For the psychoanalyst, dreaming defined by content occurs in both wake and sleep. For one group, dreaming is a state of consciousness. For the other, dreaming is a form or type of thought. For some dreaming is a biological state—REM sleep. For others a dream is an unfulfilled wish, and sometimes even a message from God.

**Table 1.1** Definitions for dreaming—a classification system paradigm

A definition of dream has three characteristic continua:
**Wake/Sleep** (a), **Recall** (b), and **Content** (c):

(a) *Sleep    Sleep Onset    Dreamlike States    Routine Waking    Alert Wake*
_____*_____*_____*_____*_____*_____

(b) *No Recall    Recall    Content    Associative Content    Written Report    Behavior*
_____*_____*_____*_____*_____*_____*_____

(c) *Awareness    Day-Reflective    Imagery    Narrative    Illogic    Bizarre/Hallucinatory*
_____*_____*_____*_____*_____*_____

Rene Descartes, a discoverer of the scientific method (a feat he attributed to a series of dreams), pointed out in 1641, "Now the principle and most frequent error that can be found in judgments consists in the fact that I judge that the ideas, which are in me, are similar to, or in conformity with certain things outside me."[27] The definition of dream differs for each individual. Some definitions contradict others. Dream research and literature purportedly addressing the same topic became conflated and confused, as adherents addressed totally different topics of study. Due to this confusion, and the inability of experts to agree or accept one overriding definition for dreaming, a consensus group was organized at the turn of the millennium, including experts as diverse as artists, writers, medical physicians, neuroscientists, psychologists, and therapists working with dreams. This group developed a multivariate classification system for dream definitions (Table 1.1).[28] Writers and researchers in the field of dream science are now asked to define their topic of discussion so that their data can be compared to that of other workers using the same definition. But dreams remain interpersonal and unique experiences, so that many knowing personally what they think a dream is, presume that it is the same for others. Many authors still avoid the thorny question of definition, and dreaming, particularly when addressed from outside the field, is often undefined.[29]

## THE PHENOMENOLOGY OF DREAMS

One approach that can be used to avoid the difficulty of definition when addressing a poorly defined topic is to limit the study to the associated and describable characteristics of the state (the phenomenology). Researchers can avoid defining "dream" and focus on measurable factors (variables) known to be associated with the state. The presumption is that if enough subjects are included, any variability in response as based on different definitions and perspectives will not significantly affect the results of a study. When studying dreams, the variables most often addressed in this manner are dream recall, dream content, and the effects dreams are reported to have on waking behavior.

Dream recall frequency is the best described of any of the measurable factors affecting dreaming. Many studies demonstrate consistent findings, making this research somewhat unusual for the dream field. The variables consistently affecting dream recall include sleep stage, time since awakening, gender, age, interest in dreaming, and dream intensity or salience.[14]

Dream content includes the visual images, associative and day-reflective memories, and emotions that are typically present in almost all dreams. Content can be difficult to study since there are a huge number of difficult to control variables known to affect the content of dream reports. Dream content is altered by type of collection (diary, interview, retrospective report), the methodology of collection (site (home vs lab), age and gender of collector, other transference factors), expectations (perceived definition of dream by subject or researcher, training), and bias (expected outcome of study by either subject or researcher). A massive psychoanalytic literature addressed dream content. However, few of these studies used scientific methodology. Almost all are anecdotal, intensely directed studies of one individual. Many suggest that there is typical dream content associated with a specific psychiatric diagnosis. Eventually, however, when studies were methodologically designed to control for competing and distracting variables, most of what had been perceived psychoanalytically as characteristic patterns for dream content turned out not to be present. In such controlled studies, the only variables that were consistently found to affect reported dream content were waking experience and gender.[4] There continue to be studies addressing the association of dream content with different psychiatric diagnoses, however none of these studies takes into account the known effects of an individual's waking experience (continuity) on dream content.[30] Dreams are clearly contiguous with an individual's waking experience. Due to such continuity, it is unsurprising that depressed individuals might have melancholic dreams of suicide, or that psychotic individuals have dreams with aberrant thoughts. It is extremely difficult to control for continuity, and few of the studies insinuating that aberrant dreaming somehow causes psychiatric illness, acknowledge its likely effects.

Many individuals use their dreams to affect their waking behaviors. We are most likely to use our dreams for decision-making, particularly in relationships and in developing attitudes towards self and others.[31] Dreams and nightmares affect next-day mood, generally in the positive direction, except in patients with PTSD. This finding indicates that dreams and nightmares are likely to have functional roles in the processing of emotions, particularly the negative emotions experienced after trauma.[32] Since dreams are often used in creative processes, presenting alternative answers to artistic and even scientific conundrums, it is those individuals who function creatively in their waking world who are those most likely to use their dreams and nightmares.[5]

Studies approach the phenomenology of dreaming by using constrained, tightly defined methodologies, so their results can be compared to other studies addressing the same topic. This approach can be used to avoid the need to define the topic under consideration. The requirement becomes one of using the same systems of methodological analysis, and the same validated questionnaire scales in a repeated and tightly defined pattern. This psychological and behavioral approach can only work, however, when the methodology is well described, the number of subjects high, and the hypothesis of the researcher is tightly constrained. Unfortunately, in a field of study such as dream, many expostulate and extend their findings as having meaning for the entire spectrum of dream definitions (including dream − undefined).

## PARTIAL METAPHORS

Humans dream. Only a human, the ones who define dreaming, can tell us whether or not she or he is dreaming. The definition paradigm (Table 1.1) was made for humans, in an attempt to be inclusive of all of the potential human definitions for dream. Many of us believe that animals dream, particularly those animals that are our pets. The definition paradigm is designed to take that possibility into account. We are prone to describing much that is important in our life experience as being "like a dream." Dreams can be viewed as such "pictured metaphors" so that images in metaphor become the stuff of dreams.[33,34] Bert States described dreams as: "images and narratives based on human experience...analogies, metaphors or models of memory structures."[35] Metaphor can be used as Aristotle suggested, "to use metaphor well is to discern similarities (to see, and/or analytically get beneath the skin of something)."[7] Yet, for dreams, comprised of many and diverse metaphors, the metaphors that we use for specific descriptions are most often misleading, describing only limited aspects of the state. Dreams can be described as visions or hallucinations. And while they have aspects of both, they are more than either. Dreams can be viewed as degraded thoughts, and sometimes as terrifying images of the night. Such metaphors can also be viewed as partial definitions.

## THE DREAMS OF MACHINES?

A further anthropomorphic step is required if we are to consider the possibility of dreaming or dream-like mentation in artificially created cognition systems. We are active creators of our machines, and we interact with our creations. We program them to address our concerns, and in that programming and interaction, they assume many of our characteristics. That interaction is not unidirectional. When we play computer games, and then go to sleep, we dream of those experiences. When we research topics of interest on the web, we follow a different course and end up in a different place with a different mindset than we would if we had not integrated ourselves into that interactive search engine. This is an active integration that changes our machines as well as changing us.

In our modern world, almost anything that can be technically described can be artificially created. We construct our dreams on a framework of brain-based visual imagery, memories, and emotions produced nonperceptually and coded as representational images in neurologic/cognitive space.[3] But is there something more to dreaming? Is the association between humans and dreaming more than a tautology? Is there something inherently special about our human capacity to dream? These are the type of questions addressed in studies of mind, philosophy, and metaphysics; topics rarely addressed by neuroscientists or the programmers and technicians developing computer AI systems. We may decide to ignore that which we consider beyond our capacity for understanding or that which we consider unacceptable. But a rational consideration of the capacity of machines to dream might be a useful intellectual endeavor, if only it brings us to further consider our human ability to dream, and what it might mean. Today we are creating AI systems that function more like the human CNS. These systems are being built using flexible and fuzzy programming logics designed to exert looser internal and external controls of processing outcomes. Such systems are utilizing new hardware formats that have neural, analogue, and quantum flexibility. Systems such as the Internet can no longer be characterized as purely software or hardware. The Internet that we use as a repository for our experiences, hopes, and dreams, is now an independent conglomerate system of inter-connected computer nodes that as an overall entity can never be turned off. Unprogrammed artificial constructs of the human CNS are currently in the process of development. In creating such systems, just what are we creating? And if some of the processing and logic in these systems is becoming equivalent to dreaming, once we have shared and delegated that capacity to our machines, just what is to become of us?

## Notes

1. Anthropomorphism can be a critique and even an insult. It can also be a stance and even an aspect of persistent belief in human potential. The philosophy of such a stance will be addressed more fully in Chapter 11. Webster's (1996). *New universal unabridged dictionary*. New York: Barnes & Noble Books.
2. Psychoanthropology is in some ways a new science. In other ways it is quite old, owing much to Plato and his humanly defining parable of the Cave. Curtis, G. (2006). *The cave painters: Probing the mysteries of the worlds finest artists*. New York: Anchor Books; Lewis-Williams, J. D. (2002). *The mind in the cave: Consciousness and the origins of art*. London and New York: Thames and Hudson; Clottes, J., & Lewis-Williams, J. D. (1998). *The shamans of prehistory: Trance and magic in the painted caves*. New York: Harry N. Abrams.
3. This book is written primarily from the perspective of Dream Science, and those who are interested are referred to this author's previous publications that address sleep and dreams (172 and counting at this point). His most recent book addresses the general status of the field and what remains of its science after its long flirtation psychoanalysis and then with the concept that REM sleep might equal dreaming. Tl, J. F. (2014). *Dream science: Exploring the forms of consciousness*. Amsterdam and Boston, MA: Academic Press (Elsevier).
4. From within the field of Dream Science, there were only a few who well able to maintain scientific rationality when faced with the monetary, political power, and belief of those proselytizing and staking their considerable reputations on the belief that REM sleep was dreaming. In the end Bill's persistence and structured research methodologies demonstrated that in the end evidence does matter. Domhoff, G. W. (2003). *The scientific study of dreams: Neural networks, cognitive development, and content analysis*. Washington, DC: American Psychological Association.
5. Pagel, J. F., Kwiatkowski, C. F., & Broyles, K. (1999). Dream use in film making. *Dreaming, 9*(4), 247–296; Pagel, J. F., Kwiatkowski, C. F. (2003). Creativity and dreaming: Correlation of reported dream incorporation into awake behavior with level and type of creative interest. *Creativity Research Journal, 15*(2&3), 199–205.
6. Buckley, K. (2009). *Dreaming and the world's religions*. New York: New York University Press. An excellent survey.
7. In Aristotle's Rhetoric as translated and interpreted by Eco, U. (1984). *Semiotics and the philosophy of language*. Bloomington, IN: Indiana University Press.
8. Pagel, J. F., & Myers, P. (2002). Definitions of dreaming: A comparison of definitions of dreaming utilized by different study populations (college psychology students, sleep lab patients, and medical professionals). *Sleep, 25*, A299–A300.
9. Homer (fl. 850 B.C.). The Odyssey, The Harvard Classics. 1909–14, Cambridge, MA.

10. Freud, S. (1953). The interpretation of dreams. In S. James (Ed.), *The standard editions of the complete psychological works of Sigmund Freud* (Vols. IV and V). London: Hogarth Press.
11. Freud, S. (1951). *Beyond the pleasure principle* (Vol. 18, J. Strachey, Trans. & Ed., The Standard Edition). London: Hogarth (Original work published 1916).
12. Nielsen, T. (2003). A review of mentation in REM and NREM sleep: "covert" REM sleep as a possible reconciliation of two opposing models. In E. Pace-Schott, M. Solms, M. Blagrove, & S. Harnad (Eds.), *Sleep and dreaming: Scientific advances and reconsiderations* (pp. 59−74). Cambridge and New York: Cambridge University Press. One of the final attempts to save REM sleep equals dreaming by postulating that whenever dreams are reported, REM sleep must be present, no matter what the recording technology indicates.
13. Foulks, D. (1985). *Dreaming: A cognitive-psychological analysis*. Hillsdale, NJ: Lawrence Erlbaum Associates. Foulks is in many ways the father of modern rational dream science.
14. Goodenough, D. (1991). Dream recall: History and current status of the field. In S. J. Ellman & J. S. Antrobus (Eds.), *The mind in sleep*. New York: John Wiley & Sons, Inc.; Kuiken, D., & Sikora, S. (1993). The impact of dreams on waking thoughts and feelings. In A. Moffitt, M. Kramer, & R. Hoffman (Eds.), *The functions of dreaming* (pp. 419−476). Albany, NY: State University of New York Press.
15. Descartes, R. (1980). *Meditations on first philosophy* (D. Cress, Trans.). Indianapolis, IN: Hackett (Original work published 1641).
16. Dement, W., & Vaughan, C. (2000). *The promise of sleep*. New York: Dell Trade Paperback. Bill was among those who discovered REM sleep. He founded the field of Sleep Medicine. In those early years, sleep was the province of psychology and psychiatry was an aspect of dreaming. Today sleep is the province of the pulmonologist, and as such, the field has only a minimal interest in the cognitive state of dreaming.
17. Hobson, J., Pace-Schott, E., & Stickgold, R. (2003). Dreaming and the brain: Toward a cognitive neuroscience of conscious states. In E. Pace-Schott, M. Solms, M. Blagrove, & S. Harnad (Eds.), *Sleep and dreaming: Scientific advances and reconsiderations* (pp. 1−50). Cambridge: Cambridge University Press; Hobson, J. (2011). *Dream life: An experimental metaphor*. Cambridge, MA: MIT Press. Allan Hobson has put a life-time of effort into defending his neuroconsciousness theory of activation-synthesis.
18. Crick, F., & Mitchenson, G. (1983). The function of dream sleep. *Nature, 304*, 111−114; Pace-Schott, E. F. (2003). Postscript: Recent findings on the neurobiology of sleep and dreaming. In E. F. Pace-Schott, M. Solms, M. Blagrove, & S. Harnard (Eds.), *Sleep and dreaming: Scientific advances and reconsiderations* (pp. 335−350). Cambridge: Cambridge University Press. Proof that reputation (a Nobel prize for discovering the DNA helix) does not necessarily extend into an ability to cogently understand a field outside your area of expertise.
19. Solms, M. (1997). *The neuropsychology of dreams: A clinico-anatomical study*. Mahwah, NJ: Lawrence Erlbaum Associates; Solms, M., & Turnbull, O. (2002). *The brain and the inner world: An introduction to the neuroscience of subjective experience* (pp. 141−143). New York: Other Press. Working in South Africa and at Anna Freud in London, and after his famous debate with Hobson at Towards a Science of Consciousness in Tucson, Mark Solms was able to publicly change the course of Dream Science.
20. Pagel, J. F. (2011). REMS and dreaming−historical perspectives. In B. N. Mallick, S. R. Pandi Perumal, R. W. McCarley, & A. R. Morrison (Eds.), *Rapid eye movement sleep: Regulation and function* (pp. 1−14). Cambridge and New York: Cambridge University Press. I find it amazing that Robert McCarley, co-author with Hobson of the activation-synthesis hypothesis would ask me to lead off his book with a chapter on the lack of association between REM sleep and dreaming.

21. Gregory, R. (1987). Dreaming. In R. L. Gregory & O. L. Zangwill (Eds.), *The Oxford companion to the mind* (pp. 201–203). New York: Oxford University Press.
22. Stickgold, R., Malia, A., Fosse, R., Propper, R., & Hobson, J. A. (2001). Brain-mind states: I. Longitudinal field study of sleep/wake factors influencing mentation report length. *Sleep, 24,* 171–179.
23. Voss, U., Holzmann, R., Tuin, I., Hobson, J. A. (2009). Lucid dreaming: A state of consciousness with features of both waking and non-lucid dreaming. *Sleep, 32,* 1191–1200. It is amazing that a study could be published by a major scientific journal in this day and age that included only three subjects in the study.
24. Pagel, J. (2013). Lucid dreaming as sleep offset waking. *Sleep, 34,* Abstract supplement.
25. The Impossible Dream (The Quest) (1964) lyrics by Joe Darion, and music by Mitch Leigh, From Dale Wasserman "Man of La Mancha".
26. Foulks, D. (1993). Data constraints on theorizing about dream function. In A. Moffit, M. Kramer, & R. Hoffmann (Eds.), *The functions of dreaming* (pp. 11–20). Albany, NY: SUNY Press.
27. Descartes, R. (1641). Objections against the meditations and replies. In J. M. Adler (Ed.), *Great books of the Western world.* Chicago, IL: Encyclopedia Britannica Inc.
28. Pagel, J. F. (Chair), Blagrove, M., Levin, R., States, B., Stickgold, B., & White, S. (2001). Defining dreaming: A paradigm for comparing disciplinary specific definitions of dream. *Dreaming, 11*(4), 195–202. And who said that philosophy was unnecessary for a scientist?
29. Pagel, J. (1999). A dream can be gazpacho. *Dreamtime, 16*(1), 6–8; Pagel, J. F., & Myers, P. (2002). Definitions of dreaming: A comparison of definitions of dreaming utilized by different study populations (college psychology students, sleep lab patients, and medical professionals). *Sleep, 25,* A299–A300. Unfortunately, there are still many studies that do not define their topic of discussion.
30. Kramer, M. (2007). *The dream experience: A systematic exploration.* New York: Routledge. Milt Kramer was among the first to try and insist that dream studies should control for bias, and have methodological and statistical consistency.
31. Pagel, J. F., & Vann, B. (1992). The effects of dreaming on awake behavior. *Dreaming, 2*(4), 229–237. Ernest Hartmann at Dreaming published this work from a young doctor practicing medicine in the middle of the Pacific Ocean.
32. Zadra, A., & Donderi, D. (2000). Nightmares and bad dreams: Their prevalence and relationship to well-being. *Journal of Abnormal Psychology, 109,* 273–281; Levin, R., & Nielsen, T. (2007). Disturbed dreaming, posttraumatic stress disorder, and affect distress: A review and neurocognitive model. *Psychological Bulletin, 133,* 482–528.
33. Hartmann, E. (1994). Nightmares and other dreams. In M. Kryger, T. Roth, & W. Dement (Eds.), *Principles and practice of sleep medicine* (2nd ed., pp. 407–410). London: W. B. Saunders; Hartmann, E. (1998). Nightmare after trauma as a paradigm for all dreams: A new approach to the nature and functions of dreaming. *Psychiatry, 61,* 223–238. There is not an area of Dream Science that Ernest Hartmann did not at sometime consider. His 1994 book inspired several generations of scientists to enter the field including this author.
34. Pagel, J. F. (2008). *The limits of dream: A scientific exploration of the mind/brain interface.* Oxford: Academic Press. This was my first book addressing the limits of Dream Science. It's a beautiful little work of which I am quite proud.
35. States, B. (1997). *Seeing in the dark: Reflections on dreams and dreaming* (p. 215). New Haven, NJ: Yale University Press. Bill was a professor of dramatic arts at UC Irvine willing to take on both Harvard and dreaming. His books are beautifully written.

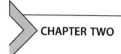

# CHAPTER TWO

# The Mechanics of Human Consciousness

*Il n'y a pas de hors-texte.*

*Derrida J. (1967)* **Of Grammatology.**

Alternative translations:

1. there is nothing outside the text;
2. there is nothing outside context;
3. unnumbered pages are part of the text.[1]

Consciousness is even more difficult to define and study than dream. It includes a wide spectrum of cognition extending from states in which we are barely aware, and barely alive, to states that are startlingly intense and remarkably focused. Consciousness is often described as the subjective component of the objective quality of experience—how we feel about ourselves and the external world. In humans, it can be viewed as a meta-state: "the experience of experiencing, the knowledge of knowing, the sense of sensing."[2] Constructing a definition has been remarkably difficult since consciousness tends to be so frustratingly intangible, as noted in the International Dictionary of Psychology:

> *Consciousness:*
>
> *The having of perceptions, thoughts and feelings; awareness. The term is impossible to define except in terms that are unintelligible without a grasp of what consciousness means. Many fall into the trap of confusing consciousness with self-consciousness—to be conscious it is only necessary to be aware of the external world. Consciousness is a fascinating but elusive phenomenon: it is impossible to specify what it is, what it does, or why it evolved. Nothing worth reading has been written about it.[3]*

While a general, all-inclusive definition for consciousness remains elusive, in the medical profession the attempt to care for an ill patient with wandering and changing awareness, consciousness must be defined

*Machine Dreaming and Consciousness.*
DOI: http://dx.doi.org/10.1016/B978-0-12-803720-1.00002-5

concretely. Clinically, consciousness is defined as an individual's arousability in response to (usually aversive) stimuli. Consciousness is sometimes restricted to specific cognitive capacities such as the ability to introspect or report one's mental status. In some writings, "consciousness" is synonymous with "self-consciousness." This perspective excludes consideration of the consciousness of others and the external world outside oneself. Consciousness is sometimes considered to be synonymous with awareness, or as the ability to focus attention or voluntarily control one's behavior. Sometimes the term "being conscious of something" has the same meaning as "to know about something."[4]

Consciousness has also been defined in a concrete, almost mechanical fashion as "information processing." Viewed as biological information processing, consciousness is a major metacognitive component of almost all brain function.[5] Consciousness is sometimes described as the global workplace of CNS information processing, "The major way in which the central nervous system adapts to novel, challenging and informative events in the world."[6] Most current theories of consciousness accept that in the human, an intimate relationship exists between consciousness and the brain. Today, many researchers, theorists, and reductive/functional philosophers take it for granted that future advances in neuroscience will demonstrate that consciousness is a state of brain functioning.

Consciousness has, however, been defined in many different ways. A survey of attempts made to address the definition of consciousness, by some of our best and brightest philosophers and scientists, is presented in Table 2.1.

A definition is in its most basic form a metaphor. Consciousness as a global state approaches the concept of absolute metaphor—an experience known to exist but otherwise impossible to define.[6] In our epistemologies, we have established many such absolutes so that such indefinable paradoxes lie at the conceptual basis of many areas of knowledge that we presume to understand. In a form that can be applied to almost any basic concept humans have chosen to define, including consciousness, Derrida eloquently captures that understanding: "Il n'y a pas de hors-texte." There is the text, and what is outside the text. And there is the page on which nothing has yet to be written. Paradoxically, integrated within the cognitive process of the reader, they are all, actually, the same.[1]

**Table 2.1** Definitions and explanations of consciousness

| | |
|---|---|
| Consciousness is the essence of Atman, a primal immanent self that is ultimately identified with Brahman—a pure transcendental, subject-object-less state that underlies and provides the ground of being for both man and nature (Upanishads) | Approx. 1000 BC. Sen, S. (2008). The vedic-upanisadic concept of Brahman. In A. Eshleman (Ed.), *Readings in philosophy of religion: East meets west* (pp. 43–51). Malden, MA: Blackwell. |
| What is (inanimate) is unaware, while what is (animate) is not unaware of undergoing change. | Aristotle, Approx. 400 BC. Shute, C. (1941). *The psychology of Aristotle: An analysis of the living being. Morningside heights* (pp. 115–118). New York: Columbia University Press. |
| While a person is asleep, the critical activities, which include thinking, sensing, recalling and remembering, do not function as they do during wakefulness. | |
| Thinking defines consciousness. A nonthinking, nondreaming state is neither conscious nor alive. | Descartes, R. (1980). *Meditations on first philosophy* (D. Cress, Trans.). Indianapolis, IN: Hackett (Original work published 1641). |
| All consciousness is consciousness of something. | Kant, I. (1929). *Critique of pure reason* (N. Kemp Smith, Trans.). London (Original work published 1781). |
| In order to be beautiful, everything must be conscious. | Nietzsche, F. (1993). *The birth of tragedy, or: Hellenism and pessimism* (S. Whiteside, Trans.). Penguin Classics (Original work published 1886). |
| The conscious sense of a coherent self is not the outcome of a distinct system in the brain. Rather, consciousness emerges from the operation of the association cortices. | Jackson, J. (1915). On affections of speech from diseases of the brain. *Brain, 38,* 107–174. |
| Scientific points of view, according to which my existence is a moment of the world's, are always naïve and at the same time dishonest, because they take for granted, without explicitly mentioning, it, the other point of view, namely that of consciousness, through which from the outset a world forms itself round me and begins to exist for me. | Merleau-Ponty, M. (1958). *Phenomenology of perception* (p. ix; C. Smith, Trans.). New York: Routledge Classics (Original work published 1945). |

*(Continued)*

**Table 2.1**  (Continued)

| | |
|---|---|
| One would not need to pose the psychological problem of an act of consciousness (prise de conscience); instead one would analyze the function and transformation of a body of knowledge. | Foucault, M. (2002). *The archaeology of knowledge* (pp. 214–215; A. Smith, Trans.). London: Routledge (Original work published 1972). |
| Consciousness is awareness resulting from the brain's functioning. | Tart, C. (1972). *States of consciousness.* New York: E.P. Dutton. |
| A process in which information about multiple individual modalities of sensation and perception is combined into a unified multidimensional representation of the state of the system and its environment, and integrated with information about memories and the needs of the organism, generating emotional reactions and programs of behavior to adjust the organism to the environment... | Thatcher, R. W., & John, E. R. (1977). *Foundations of cognitive processes* (p. 294). Hillsdale, NJ: Lawrence Erlbaum Associates. |
| We can not form more than a schematic conception between facts and conceptual schemes or systems of representation. | Nagel, T. (1979). What is it like to be a bat? In *Mortal questions* (p. 171). Cambridge: Cambridge University Press. |
| In our naiveté, it seems now that conscious states are a single, unified natural kind of brain state, but we should consider the possibility that the brain is fitted with a battery of monitoring systems, with varying ranges of activity, and with varying degrees of efficiency, where consciousness may be but one amongst others, or where these systems cross-classify what we now think of conscious states. States we now group together as conscious states may no more constitute a natural kind than does say, dirt, or gems, or things-that-go-bump-in-the-night. | Churchland, P. S. (1983). Consciousness: The transmutation of a concept. *Pacific Philosophical Quarterly, 64,* 92. |
| ...a matter not of arrival at a point but rather a matter of a representation exceeding some threshold of activation over the whole cortex or large parts thereof. | Dennett, D. (1991). *Consciousness explained* (p. 166). Boston, MA: Little, Brown & Co. |

*(Continued)*

**Table 2.1** (Continued)

| | |
|---|---|
| Consciousness is at once the most immediately present and the most inscrutably intangible entity in human existence. | Norretranders, T. (1991). *The user illusion* (p. ix). New York: Viking. |
| We can talk to each other about consciousness, but it is fundamentally, ineradicably experienced only alone, from within. | |
| Consciousness is the experience of experiencing, the knowledge of knowing, the sense of sensing. | |
| We believe that it is hopeless to try to solve the problems of consciousness by general philosophical arguments: what is needed are new suggestions for experience that might throw light on these problems. (p. 19) | Crick, F. (1994). *The astonishing hypothesis: The scientific search for the soul.* New York: Charles Scribner's Sons. |
| 1. Not all the operations of the brain correspond to consciousness. 2. Consciousness involves some form of memory, probably a very short term one. 3. Consciousness is closely associated with attention. (p. 15) | |
| The subject matter is perhaps best characterized as "the subjective quality of experience." When we perceive, think, and act, there is a while of causation and information processing, but this processing does not usually go on in the dark. There is also an internal aspect; there is something it feels like to be a cognitive agent. This internal aspect is conscious experience. | Chambers, D. (1996). *The conscious mind: In search of a fundamental theory* (p. 4). New York: Oxford University Press. |
| …it is not possible to give a definition of "consciousness"… | Searle, J. R. (1998). *The rediscovery of the mind.* Cambridge, MA: The MIT Press. |
| What I mean by "consciousness" can best be illustrated by examples. When I wake up from a dreamless sleep, I enter a state of consciousness, a state that continues so long as I am awake. When I go to sleep or am put under general anesthetic or die, my conscious states cease. If during sleep I have dreams, I become conscious… | |

*(Continued)*

**Table 2.1** (Continued)

| | |
|---|---|
| Consciousness, as we commonly think of it, from its basic levels to the most complex, is the unified mental pattern that brings together the object and self. (p. 11) | Damasio, A. (1999). *The feeling of what happens: Body and emotion in the making of consciousness.* San Diego, CA: Harcourt, Inc. |
| I propose that we become conscious when the organism's representative devices exhibit a specific kind of wordless knowledge—the knowledge that the organisms own state has been changed by an object—and when such knowledge occurs along with the salient representation of an object. (p. 25) | |
| The consciousness of the mind is the combined result of the electrical activity of the brain. | Blaha, S. (2000). *Cosmos and consciousness* (p. 253). New Hampshire: Price Hill Publishing. |
| Consciousness is the crutch of cognitive neuroscience, perhaps the most widely used covert tool for the classification of mental phenomena. Yet this frequently used hypernym does not even have a definition. Is it a product, a process, or a thing? There is not even good agreement what the theory about consciousness would be like. | Buzsaki, G. (2006). *Rhythms of the brain* (p. 360). Oxford: Oxford University Press. |
| Consciousness in the field of engineering is not "something" which can be emulated artificially. Consciousness is not a thing which must be put into a machine. Consciousness is not an emergent property stemming out from complexity. | Tagliasco, V. (2007). Artificial consciousness—A technological discipline. In A. Chella & R. Manzotti (Eds.), *Artificial consciousness* (p. 21). Charlottesville, VA: Imprint Academic. |
| An artificial conscious being would be a being which appears to be conscious because (it) acts and behaves as a conscious human being. | |
| A person, or other entity, is conscious if they experience something; conversely, if a person or entity experiences nothing they are not conscious. | Velmans, M. (2009). How to define consciousness—and how not to define consciousness. *Journal of Consciousness Studies, 16,* 139–156. |

*(Continued)*

**Table 2.1** (Continued)

| | |
|---|---|
| A process can be said to be conscious: (1) in the sense that one is conscious of the process, (2) in the sense that the operation of the process is accompanied by consciousness, and (3) in the sense that consciousness enters into or causally influences the process. | |
| We will refrain from trying to give a universal definition of consciousness; for AI-development the definition does not have to be universal, or applicable to humans for explanation of human consciousness...we define consciousness as the ability to "rise above programming." | Williams, H. (2012). *Why we need "conscious artificial intelligence"*. Available from http://mindconstruct. com/webpages/newsiem/25. Accessed 21.07.15. |

## HUMAN CONSCIOUSNESS

It is humans who describe consciousness. In order to address the question of the potential for consciousness in our artificial creations, we first need to consider consciousness in humans. Human consciousness is not a unitary, all-encompassing, or specifically defined state. Consciousness clearly exists in different forms. Different forms are present in both wake and sleep. Forms of waking consciousness include at least the following: focused waking, self-referential (default) waking, creative waking, drowsy waking, hypnosis, focused meditation, unfocused meditation, and a wide spectrum of alternative states that can be induced by drugs, music, exercise, dance, and ecstatic trance.[7] During waking, states of consciousness flux and change across the day. A majority of our time is spent in various forms of self-referential or default consciousness, mind-wandering tasks such as autobiographical memory retrieval, envisioning possible futures, and conceiving the perspectives of others.[8]

Sleep is considered to be a conscious state because of reports of dreaming—mentation reported as occurring during those states. Some neuroscientists, specifically, Francis Crick and Cristof Koch, have expressed their doubts as to the presence of consciousness in sleep. Yet they have difficulty accounting for dreaming, particularly when that dreaming occurring during REMS: "It seems likely that the essential features of consciousness are probably not usually present in slow wave sleep, nor under a deep anesthetic. Rapid eye movement (REM) or dreaming sleep is another matter. It seems that a limited form of consciousness occurs in REM sleep."[9] The forms of sleeping consciousness are most often categorized based on their sleep stage of origin. While there are those who believe that sleep can be a nonconscious state, there are far more data supporting the possibility that forms of consciousness, most reported on waking as dreams, are present throughout sleep.

In the human, consciousness is not just one state, but a rapidly changing and fluxing state of cognitive integration that changes phenomenologically across the day and night. Different forms of consciousness occur in wake, during sleep, and on the borderline between waking and sleeping consciousness. Behaviorally each state differs in the degree of perceptual isolation, type of thought processing, level of attention, memory access, social teachability, and level of conscious control. These characteristics can be used to describe the spectrum of these varyingly well-defined states of consciousness (Table 2.2). Primary differences between waking and sleeping states of consciousness include the absence of volitional control and social teachability for most of the states of sleep. The conscious states of sleep are also less likely to include focused attention as a component. Each sleep stage has characteristic dreaming activity that differs cognitively, emotionally, and visually from dreaming in the other sleep stages.[8]

## THE NEUROBIOLOGY OF HUMAN CONSCIOUSNESS

Much of what we understand of the various forms of human consciousness is based on our understanding of the biologic framework on which consciousness is built. Today most scientists, most philosophers, and most of the rest of us believe that the brain, the central nervous system, is that biologic framework. In attempting to understand the potential for consciousness to be produced by artificial constructs, it is necessary to consider if at least briefly, our current understanding of the neurobiology on which the biological constructs of consciousness might be based. The biologic components of consciousness that we understand best are the structural neuroanatomy, the neurochemistry, and the electrophysiology.

Table 2.2 Behavioral characteristics comparison between described forms of waking and sleeping consciousness

| Waking states | Perceptual isolation | Thought—attention | Memory access | Volitional control | Teachability |
|---|---|---|---|---|---|
| Focused wake | Lowest | Focused | High | High | High |
| Self-referential (default) wake | Low | Self-focused | High—associative | High | Characteristic |
| Drowsy wake | Low | Un-focused | High | High | Characteristic |
| Creative wake | Low—moderate | Focused | High—associative | High | High |
| Hypnosis | Moderate | Variable | High | Variable | Variable |
| Focused meditation | Moderate | Variable | High | High | High |
| Unfocused meditation | Moderate | Variable | High | High | High |
| *Sleeping states* | | | | | |
| Hypnogognic states (stage 1) | Moderate | Disassociated | High | Low—variable | Mod |
| Stage 2 dreaming | Moderate | Continuity | High | Low | Low |
| REM sleep dreaming | High | Focused | High | Low | Low |
| Deep sleep (stage 3) dreaming | High | Unfocused | Low | Low | None |
| Lucid dreaming | Low | Focused | High | High | Moderate |
| Sleep meditation | High | Focused | High | High | High |

## NEUROANATOMY

Even in the earliest eras of medicine and philosophy, it was clear that anatomic alterations in the brain induced by trauma and disease could produce alterations in cognitive functioning. Based on such observations, philosophers predating Aristotle concluded that the seat of consciousness was in the brain.[10] Today, the study of brain pathophysiology—whether based on illness, trauma, or surgery—continues to be a technique used to study aspects of consciousness. Blunt-force trauma to the head, neurosurgery, anoxia, electrical shock, neurotoxins, and anesthetics can induce clinical unconsciousness. What generally is described as a concussion is a short-term experience of impaired consciousness induced by head trauma. When more severe, generalized brain insult can lead to a prolonged vegetative state (coma) in which volitional control and response to external stimuli are varyingly lost for extended periods of time. Studies of such states have led us to an understanding of consciousness as an essential global state that is preferentially preserved after extensive trauma or insult to the brain.

Technology has been developed that can be used to noninvasively probe into the anatomy of neurological illness and trauma. For almost 100 years, X-rays have provided increasingly detailed insight into skull structure and radio-opaque intrusions (such as bullets). More recently, computerized tomography (CT) scans used with injected radio-sensitive markers, and magnetic resonance imaging (MRI) records of the response of magnetically aligned atomic particles to external radio waves have been used to more clearly define soft-brain neuroanatomy. Newer scanning techniques can be used to look at brain functioning as well as brain anatomy. Functional MRI (fMRI), recording areas of glucose and oxygen metabolism in metabolically active areas of the brain, and positron emission tomography (PET) recording the metabolic uptake of radioactive markers, operate on a time differential short enough so that brain activity (function) can be recorded on a real-time basis. These tools allow the technician to record the brain activity occurring in response to a stimulus or even a thought. Experimental stimuli such as visualizing the color red or thinking about God, or dogs, can be shown to produce consistent patterns of fMRI or PET activation. The confounding methodology involved in using this approach will be more fully addressed in the next chapter. However, such experiments do indicate that complex, widely separated, and individually variable CNS activity occurs in response to discrete experimental stimuli.

Specific aspects of consciousness, such as attention and directed thought, have proven amenable to evaluation using such techniques. Global aspects of mental functioning, such as consciousness, sleep, wake, and dreaming, have proven more difficult to study using scanning technologies.

## NEUROCHEMISTRY

Ancient shamans first realized the capacity of drugs to alter consciousness. Psychedelic plants and fungi are among the first neurochemicals utilized by our species. Psychoactive drugs were incorporated into ritual and religion. Eventually, altered states of consciousness and their negative effects became a societal concern rather than part of a process of religious initiation. The study of such compounds evolved into the field of neurochemistry. Various milder chewable and smokeable neuroactive agents such as betel, coca, caffeine, marijuana, opiates, and tobacco have a long history of use that continues in todays' mainstream society as well as in modern-era hunter-gathering groups. Archeologically, the societal development of agriculture marks the advent of ethanol (grain–based alcohol)—also in continued heavy use.

Neurocognitive effects and side effects are the most common drug actions induced by the many agents in today's medical pharmacopeia. Sedation is the most commonly induced effect, however, agitation and insomnia are also quite common. Until quite recently, these symptoms were viewed as global, affecting the entire CNS. In the last 50 years, however, a wide spectrum of neurotransmitters and neuromodulators have been described that affect the activity and intercommunication of nerve cells. Almost all pharmacological agents alter the activity of one or another of these agents producing changes in CNS alertness with sedation or stimulation as effects or side effects. These neurotransmitters and neuromodulators are the chemical modulators of consciousness.

## ELECTROPHYSIOLOGY

In the early 20th century, electroencephalography (EEG) analysis was developed as a technique for recording brain-based electrical fields. Today EEGs are used in the clinical setting to diagnose seizure disorders, for polysomnographic sleep staging, and to determine the presence or absence of brain neural activity after cerebral insult. The absence of such activity is legally utilized in defining the absence of consciousness, what is sometimes referred to as death. The origin of these EEG signals remains a topic of debate in the field. After the discovery that it is an electrochemical interface at the cell membrane that allows nerve cells to develop spike potentials (fire) and transmit electric signals over cellular processes and across synapses in transmission line fashion to the next cells, it was deemed logical that the EEG should reflect the activity of these neurological spike potentials. However, it has been difficult to describe how individual, discrete spike potentials might contribute to forming the propagated synchronous global EEG rhythms that typically occur during sleep.[11]

These frequency-based extraneural electrical fields affect neuron activity at the neural membrane. Neurochemicals and electrical fields induce an interconnected dance affecting the tendency of the cells to fire, seting ionic equilibrium states, and supplying energy for cellular functions. Specific frequencies are linked to chemical metabolic oscillators at the neural membrane inducing a reciprocal rhythmatic opening and closing of ionic gateways and channels (potassium for alpha frequency, calcium for sigma frequency). This fluxing system affects the tendency of neurons to fire, resets cellular equilibrium, affects signal-to-noise ratio, acts in neural communication, and alters cellular messaging systems. In the CNS, these synchronous electrical fields can be utilized in producing integration between widely spaced neuronal populations.[12] Since this system affects the electrically sensitive neuro-messaging systems at the neural cell membrane, it has the potential to affect expression and access to memory systems, including electrically sensitive cellular DNA.[13] Today, magnetoencephalography (MEG) denotes the limits of electrophysiological research. Faster than fMRI and PET, MEG can be used to chart the rapid flux of these highly multivariate fields as they topographically flux and globally change on a millisecond-to-millisecond timescale across the CNS.[14]

## HUMAN CONSCIOUSNESS—AN OVERVIEW OF THE PROCESSING SYSTEM

Our functional human capacity to hold and maintain data is quite limited. We are typically able to retain less than 10 (3—7 based on study and population) unrelated words or symbols in our working memory.[15] It is our capacity for metacognitive consciousness (an awareness and understanding of our own thought processes) that allows us to function in complex external and internal environments. There we are able integrate, metaphorically compare, and process masses of perceptual, memiotic, behavioral, and emotional data. We can exist and operate in multiple and complex versions of consciousness simultaneously (e.g., driving the car, planning our weekend, extending relationships, chewing gum, and exploring the cognitive extent of consciousness, all while using extender devices such as our radio and cell phones to communicate with a machine database and other humans). We understand little of our own capacity for consciousness. But most evidence indicates that the biological framework for consciousness is global. No specific chemical, electrophysiologic, or neuroanatomic switch has been discovered that can turn our capacity for consciousness on and off.

## CONSTRUCTING MACHINE CONSCIOUSNESS

While consciousness is difficult to define, in a biological system such as our own there is strong evidence that consciousness develops within a global workspace, a CNS framework constructed of anatomy, chemistry, and electrical fields.[16] Computer systems are programmed from the perspective of our own consciousness to contribute to and help to support our own process of cognitive integration. The data entered are based on our own ability to understand what various information might mean. We process those data using scientific, mathematical, and logical logarithms and formulas developed to describe our cognitive understanding of our external and internal world. The resultant integration of these applications must then be presented in a way that we as humans can understand.

Several factors circumscribe out ability to create systems of artificial consciousness that are comparable and compatible with our biologic consciousness:

1. We have only a very limited understanding of our own consciousness.
2. Our perceptual systems integrate information using human biological sensory modalities. We limit and constrain our artificial intelligence

(AI) systems to communicate with us within the limitations of these sensory modalities.

3. Currently interactions with these systems are constrained by our motor, and vocal capacities (speech, eye tracking, and keyboard).

4. Computer systems are electronic switching, chip-based, and electrically powered, systems constructed and operating in different and basic ways from the biologic anatomic, chemical, and electrophysiological framework of the CNS. Both systems, however, have the capacity to switch from digital to analog formats.

5. Computer systems operate using massive, parallel, and comparatively (to humans) massive levels of data processing. Our conscious process is one of metaphilosophical integration, metaphoric comparison, and overall, yet limited, data integration.

6. Computer systems are programmed utilizing mathematical, parametric logics. It is unclear as to whether human biologic processing systems are based on any form of set logic (i.e., humans may not have a theory of mind).

It has recently become apparent that in order for machine systems to better function in the human-defined environment, they will likely need to become more flexible and less controlled. If they are to function independently at a level equivalent and interactional with humans, they will need to have the capacity to self-learn (i.e., they need to be systems with AI). In order to create such systems, the programmer must find a way to construct an independent global cognitive workspace for the machine that will still be amenable to programmer control. Many of these systems will utilize software and hardware that attempts to parody the processing functions of the human CNS. In doing so these systems will be constrained by human logical, perceptual, and interface limitations (1—6 above).

In some ways such strong AI systems, being our creations, have more in common with our consciousness than the forms of consciousness based that we share with other animals (see Chapter 3: Animal Dreaming—Animal Consciousness). We have built our AI systems using Human philosophic, mathematical, and electronic equivalents. We have programmed them using our anthropocentric logic. Systems in current development will incorporate psuedomorphs of the biologic components of consciousness, artificial neural nets rather than cellular neurons, electrical rather than neurochemical power, and flexible/fuzzy logics rather than protein- and

DNA-based directive programming. In parodying human processing, such systems are more likely to have human-equivalent capacities for functioning in ill-defined space (i.e., they may be required for independent robotic applications). It is also more likely that they will have the capacity to develop coherent responses to exceedingly complex and sometimes apparently illogical data environments (e.g., predictions for the effects of global warming). It is also hoped that they may be able to develop creative and alternative solutions to what today seem to be apparently insolvable problems. The forms of consciousness that such systems develop will share characteristics as well as differences human consciousness. The forms of machine consciousness have many similarities with human forms of consciousness that are most often present during the sleep states—the alternative consciousnesses of dream.

## Notes

1. Derrida, J. (1967). *Of grammatology*. Paris: Les Editions de Minuit; a famously debated quote adapted in this text to address the topic of dreaming. Alternative translations: Pidgen, C. R. (1990). On a defense of Derrida. *The Critical Review, 30–32*, 40–41; Derrida (1988) Afterword, p. 136; and M. Wood (2016) London Review of Books February 4. Not everyone loves Derrida, and this, one of his most famous statements, has been critiqued as gnomic.
2. Norretranders, T. (1991). *The user illusion* (p. ix). New York: Viking.
3. Sutherland, N. S. (Ed.). (1989). *The international dictionary of psychology*. New York: Continuum.
4. Chambers, D. (1996). *The conscious mind* (pp. 3–6). Oxford: Oxford Press.
5. Block, N. (1995). On a confusion about a function of consciousness. *Journal of Consciousness Studies, 18*, 227–272.
6. Shoben, E. J. (1961). Culture, ego, psychology and an image of man. *American Journal of Psychotherapy, 15*, 395–408; Lakoff, G., & Johnson, M. (1980). *Metaphors we live by*. Chicago, IL: University of Chicago Press.
7. Krippner, S. (1972). Altered states of consciousness. In J. White (Ed.), *The highest states of consciousness* (pp. 1–5). Garden City, NY: Anchor Books. Stan survived the 1960s.
8. Pagel, J. F. (2014). *Dream science: Exploring the forms of consciousness*. Amsterdam and Boston, MA: Academic Press (Elsevier).
9. Crick, F., & Koch, C. (1992). The problem of consciousness. *Scientific American, 267*, 152–159. Crick handed off the mantle of his "reputation" in the area of neuroconsciousness to Cristof Koch who now works with the Allen Institute.
10. Gross, C. (1995). Aristotle on the brain. *The Neuroscientist, 1*(4), 245–250.
11. Christakos, C. N. (1986). The mathematical basis of population rhythms in nervous and neuromuscular systems. *International Journal of Neuroscience, 29*, 103–107.
12. Cheek, T. R. (1989). Spatial aspects of calcium signaling. *Journal of Cellular Science, 93*, 211–216.
13. Pagel, J. F. (2012). The synchronous electrophysiology of conscious states. *Dreaming, 22*, 173–191. This entire area of focus was critiqued in the early 1990s as

psuedoscince. Today, it has become generally accepted as the likely physiological platform for consciousness.

14. Steriade, M. (2001). *The intact and sliced brain*. Cambridge: MIT Press.
15. Tulving, E. (1983). *Elements of episodic memory*. Oxford: Oxford University Press; Cowan, N. (2005). *Working memory capacity*. East Sussex: Psychology Press.
16. Baars, B. J., & McGovern, K. (1996). Cognitive views of consciousness: What are the facts? How do we explain them? In M. Velmans (Ed.), *The science of consciousness: Psychological, neuropsychological, and clinical reviews* (p. 96). London: Routledge. This global workspace theory is now, perhaps, the most universally accepted biological theory of neuroconsciousness.

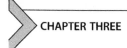

# CHAPTER THREE

# Animal Dreaming—Animal Consciousness

*If a lion could talk, we could not understand him.*

**Ludwig Wittgenstein (1958)[1]**

Dreaming and consciousness have been defined, described, and endlessly discussed by our species. Versions of each are present in our closest relatives, as well as in creatures existing on only the edge of biological existence. Consciousness and dreaming are likely quite different for those creatures which are not us.

## ANIMAL DREAMING

The Greeks of Classic Antiquity believed that animals could dream. Aristotle in "The History of Animals" wrote: "It would appear that not only do men dream, but horses also, and dogs, and oxen; aye, and sheep, and goats, and all viviparous quadrupeds; and dogs show their dreaming by barking in their sleep."[2]

Today we know that all mammals, most monotremes, and many birds experience episodes of REM sleep, a state associated in humans with a high frequency of dream recall.[3] In the last 50 years, most theories of neuroconsciousness have posited that REM sleep, this near-universal electrophysiological brain state, is the biologic marker for dreaming. If such theories are correct, animals that have REM sleep are dreaming. Yet it is rare that the complex CNS can be addressed with such simplicity. It is now quite clear that in humans REM sleep occurs without dreaming, and dreaming without REM sleep. Different forms of dream consciousness occur with each of the stages of sleep.[4]

*Machine Dreaming and Consciousness.*
DOI: http://dx.doi.org/10.1016/B978-0-12-803720-1.00003-7

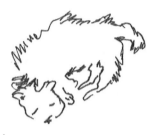

**Figure 3.1** The dreaming dog.

## PERIODIC LIMB MOVEMENTS OF SLEEP

Many of us have seen dogs and other animals make running motions, noises, and facial contortions in their sleep (Fig. 3.1). But are they actually dreaming? In humans, such sleep-associated behaviors are rarely associated with dreaming. Infants less than a year of age, make grimaces, mouth movements, and vocalizations during REM sleep (called active sleep in this age grouping), but such behaviors disappear before their first birthdays. Leg and arm movements during sleep are common in humans, but they are most often associated with unwanted behavioral activity in sleep (a parasomnia) called periodic limb movement disorder (PLMD). These repetitive movements, sometimes occurring as often as 100−200 times each hour, can severely disrupt sleep. PLMD becomes more common as we age, and is present in more than 30% of 80-year-olds. The tendency to have periodic limb movements is often inherited and is associated with a series of disorders including attention deficit/hyperactivity disorder (AD/HD) in children, renal failure, low iron levels, and the use of some medications (particularly antidepressants).[5] These limb movements can produce recurrent arousals from sleep, but they are rarely associated with reports of dreaming. Humans who make such arm and leg movements in their sleep are not dreaming of running, except perhaps, those with the unusual diagnosis of REM sleep behavior disorder.

## REM SLEEP BEHAVIOR DISORDER

REM sleep differs from the other sleep stages in three primary ways:

**1.** Eyes move repetitively back and forth with conjugate movements;

2. Scalp-recorded brain EEG activity changes from the synchronous rolling wave forms of the other stages to disorganized higher-frequency activity that resembles wake; and

3. There is a reduction of motor activity so that skeletal and facial muscles become flaccid.[3]

For the interpreting technician, REM sleep is present only when all these criteria are met.[6] During REM sleep other physiologic changes that take place include genital erections, an increased variability in heart and respiratory rates, a relaxation of gastrointestinal sphincters, and a high frequency of reported dreaming (>80%).[7] None of these, however, are required criteria that must be met in order for REM sleep to be present. For most of us, atonia (the motor block of REM sleep) means that we do not physically act out our dreams during our sleep. We are unable to move during dreaming. Individuals with REM sleep behavior disorder (RBD), however, have lost the motor block associated with REM sleep, so that they actively move during some episodes of dreaming. These individuals often present clinically with a history of sleep-associated injuries to themselves or their bed-partners. These actions are most often hitting a bedside object, or their partner, or leaping from the bed. Some RBD patients will report dreams and nightmares that include a storyline somehow related to such an action. However, as in most studies of dreaming, the story is rarely so simple. Clearly associated dream storylines such as running or hitting are present in only a minority of cases. And such an apparent acting out of dreams occurs outside REM sleep for some affected individuals.[8] It is these humans with RBD, however, who have observable nocturnal behaviors that are closest behaviorally to the apparent dreams of dogs and other animals.

## PROVING THAT DOGS DREAM

Aristole was not always correct in his closely reasoned suppositions. He contradicted early philosophers in asserting that the seat of cognition and mind was in the heart rather than the brain.[9] It is also possible that Aristotle was mistaken in making the assertion that animals dream. And if the motions he observed in dogs' sleep did indicate the presence of dreaming, it is likely that those dreams are quite different, with different functions than the dreams of humans.

If we are to know when an animal is dreaming, one commonly used approach is to document the objective presence of brain activity (REM sleep) presumably associated with dreaming. But, as noted, there is only very limited evidence that such a correlate exists. In humans dreamers can only report whether dreaming has occurred after they wake. In studying the possibility that dogs might be dreaming, the researcher does not have access to a dream report (due to the lack of language capacity to report whether or not a dream has taken place). fMRI scanning can be used to record brain activity during sleep. Some of the same brain areas are activated during periods of REM sleep as when the dog is involved in waking. This finding has been construed to prove not only that dogs are dreaming as suggested by Aristotle, but that the content of their dreams, as in humans, has continuity with their waking experience.[10] Aristotle suggested that dogs are making running motions with their legs because they are dreaming of running.[3] Based on the dream experience of an intruder, they bark. While seemingly reasonable, this assumption is based on a series of suppositions, some of which may not be true (Table 3.1).

Early theorists in the sleep field suggested that human eye movements in REM sleep might reflect the activity or experience about which the person is dreaming.[11] However, dream content studies indicate that dreams of tennis or ping-pong are a rarity, except perhaps among professional athletes in those sports. Yet, this perspective has been extended outside the dream field. Antonio Damasio (1999) concludes that animals experience self-referential dreaming: "In dream sleep, during which consciousness returns in its odd way, emotional expressions are easily detectable in humans and animals."[12] Google included this supposition as part of a commercial for its browser system. A child actor asks Google, "Do dogs dream?" The Google interface replies, "Dogs dream, and just like us, what they dream of is their waking experience."[13] As noted, the logic getting to this point is circular and full of some unfilled holes, but since it has been stated by the Google interface, a system that is apparently much more intelligent than any human, it must be true.

Whether or not you believe that animals dream, depends on the definition that you use for dreaming. Animals have brain activity that includes REM sleep and wake-like brain activation in sleep—one definition used for dreaming. There is less evidence for bizarre or hallucinatory content, metaphor, wish fulfillment, or lucid control, and there is no evidence that they are corresponding with a deity.

**Table 3.1** Evidence suggesting that other animals may not dream

1. In humans dreams are reported from all stages of sleep [REM sleep does not equal dreaming]
   a. Dream recall frequency is no higher from REM sleep than from sleep onset (>80%) with dreaming reported from almost half of awakenings from stage 2 and deep sleep (stage 3)[a]
   b. Despite the high incidence of reported dreaming, fMRI brain activity during sleep onset differs markedly from the brain activity present during REM sleep (much of the visual cortex remains activated during this stage)[b]
   c. During deep sleep very different areas of the brain are activated, yet dreaming activity is still reported[c]
   d. During other light stages of sleep (stage 2) activated areas of the cortex can include the same areas activated during REM sleep[d]
2. In the adult human, motor activities such as leg movements and vocalizations are suppressed during REM sleep (depressed voluntary motor activity defines the REM sleep state)
   a. Such behaviors are occasionally present in the rare patient with REM sleep behavior disorder (RBD) who may act out dreams with behaviors and motor activity during sleep. Approximately 50% of these individuals have RBD as a symptom associated with a progressive neurological illness—most commonly Parkinson's disease[e]
   b. Neonates and infants less than a year of age my have vocalizations and facial grimacing during REM sleep (active sleep), but this behavior disappears as early as 6 months of age.[f] In an infant, prior to the development of communication skills, there is no possibility of a dream report so it remains unclear as to whether these activities in REM sleep are associated with dreaming
   c. When originally described, Dement and others proposed that the conjugate, back-and-forth eye movements present in REM sleep were occurring secondary to dreams of tennis or ping-pong matches.[g] If this were true, parodying a dog's repetitive dream of running, the human dreams of tennis
   d. Periodic limb movements in humans resemble the dogs' "running" activity during sleep. These common repetitive leg movements in humans are more common outside REM sleep and are rarely, if ever, associated with dreaming[h]
3. No animal that is not human, has ever reported dreaming. It is possible that some of the great apes trained in symbol communication will describe dreaming if a way is found to somehow cogently convey the question. But until that point, it remains a human-based supposition that animals dream

[a]Foulks, D. (1985). *Dreaming: A cognitive-psychological analysis*. Hillsdale, NJ: Lawrence Erlbaum Associates. A classic of dream science.

[b]Oudiette, D., Dealberto, M. J., Uguccioni, G., Golmard, J. L., Merino-Andreu, M., Tafti, M., et al. (2012). Dreaming without REM sleep. *Consciousness and Cognition, 21*, 1129; Horikawa, T., Tamaki, M., Miyawaki, Y., & Kanitani, Y. (2013). Neural decoding of visual imagery during sleep. *Science, 340*, 639–642.

[c]Pagel, J. F. (2014). *Dream science: Exploring the forms of consciousness*. Amsterdam and Boston, MA: Academic Press (Elsevier).

[d]Suzuki, H. Uchiyama, M., Tagaya, H., Ozaki, H., Kuriyama, K., Aritake, S., et al. (2004). Dreaming during non-rapid eye movement sleep in the absence of prior rapid eye movement sleep. *Sleep, 27* (8), 1486–1490.

[e]Schenck, C., & Mahowald, M. (2002). REM sleep behavior disorder: Clinical, developmental and neuroscience perspectives 16 years after its formal identification in SLEEP. *Sleep, 25*, 120–138. Among the most recently discovered of significant sleep disorders.

[f]Pagel, J. F. (Ed.). (2006). Pediatric (infant and pediatric sleep) American Academy of Sleep Medicine–Training Program [video-CD].

[g]Dement, W., & Vaughan, C. (2000). *The promise of sleep*. New York: Dell Trade Paperback. The history of the sleep science field by its founder.

[h]Verma, N., & Kushida, C. (2014). Restless legs and PLMD. In J. F. Pagel & S. R. Pandi-Perumal (Eds.), *Primary care sleep disorders: A practical guide* (2nd ed., pp. 339–344). New York: Springer Press.

# THE FUNCTIONS OF DREAMING

The function of dreams in humans is a subject of continuing debate. There have always been some who believe that dreams have no function and should therefore be ignored. But almost everyone dreams. This persistence of the cognitive experience of dreaming from generation to generation since the recorded dawn of human consciousness, strongly suggests that dreams might have important functions. Almost all such evolutionarily preserved functions are preserved because they contribute in some way to improved survival. One proposed function for dreams is as threat rehearsal. In a threat rehearsal dream or nightmare, the individual experiences the dangers of the waking world without being exposed to any actual external danger of physical damage. In that alternative world alternative strategies and responses to these dangers can safely be explored.[14] If animals dream, such may still be a primary function for dreaming. This function for dreaming would have also been important for early humans who lived in a world of dangerous animals for which they were sometimes prey. But in today's technologically based world, it is not apparent as to how this function for dreaming might contribute to our increased survival. It is potential that threat rehearsal dreams are a spandral, a structure or behavior evolutionarily preserved that has no apparent function.[15] Perhaps since evolutionary change occurs slowly, there have been insufficient generations for such a genetic change to occur since humans moved away from living as hunter-gatherers on the plains of Africa. The best evidence for the persistence of this function for dreams in humans is the diagnosis of posttraumatic stress disorder (PTSD). These individuals have had waking experiences of overwhelming psychological or physical trauma. Among the most common symptoms of PTSD are intrusive re-experiences of that trauma. This is most commonly experienced as recurrent nightmares.[16]

The capacity for innovation and rapid technological change is a primary characteristic defining our species, the characteristic that differentiates us from other animals and allowed us to dominate the other races of proto-humans.[17] The capacity for innovation and creativity is in part dependent on our ability to dream. Dreaming, as an altered cognitive state from waking consciousness, allows us to explore alternative perspectives on waking reality, requiring us to organize thought in a way that differentiates our internal world from the perceptual reality of the outside world. Making variations on a theme is a crux of creative thought.[18] Dreams can be used in developing alternative approaches to waking functioning, making decisions, and answering questions.[19] Most artists and writers, many scientists, and even philosophers integrate and use their dreams in their creative process. Some of these creative dream inspirations have produced major changes in our human understanding of self and the world around us. Examples include Descarte's dream of the scientific method, Kekule's dream of the benzene ring, and Lowei's discovery of the first chemical neurotransmitter. Dream-based inspirations have a clear history of contributing to both individual and species-based creativity.[20] Some of the strongest evidence for a primary function for dreaming is in creativity.[21] Creativity has class 1 survival value (Table 3.2). Dreaming in its involvement in the creative process can be considered to have at least class 2 survival value.[22]

Dreams clearly have other functions beyond their roles in threat rehearsal-based emotional processing and creativity. Dreams provide a form of cognitive feedback, giving the organism insight into CNS processing that is occurring during sleep. Based on psychoanalytic/Freudian perspectives, dreams provide clues into the psychodynamics of the unconscious mental process.[23] Today this approach is better known for its limitations and failures in the treatment of psychiatric illness, yet psychoanalytic approaches continue to be used as an approach to self-understanding, and as an approach to the critique and understanding of art, music, and film.[24] One of the proven functions for sleep is in the incorporation of waking experiences into memory. Dreams give insight into this process.[25]

It has become popular to suggest that dreams have no function, or that if dreams do have a function, it is likely to resemble the computer process of drive defragmentation—deleting from the CNS entangled and extraneous thoughts and memories that could potentially interfere with waking functioning.[26] This theory suggests that dreams are extraneous, nonuseful thoughts, degraded forms of mentation, fragments of excess memory being purged from the CNS during sleep. This computer science-based theory of neuroconsciousness, has contributed to perspectives suggesting that dreaming is a cognitive distraction that should be ignored and deemphasized.[27]

## COMPARING ANIMAL DREAMS TO HUMAN DREAMS

Humans and animals utilize similar biologic systems for cognitive processing, a framework of approximately equivalent neuroanatomy,

**Table 3.2** Classification of functional significance for a survival characteristic

1. The characteristic has a survival characteristic at that point in development
2. The characteristic does not have a survival characteristic at that point in development, but it is necessary to build another characteristic that eventually will have high survival value
3. The characteristic does not have a survival characteristic at that point in development, but it will eventually be combined with other characteristics, the combination eventually having high survival value
4. The characteristic itself does not have a survival characteristic but it is the outcome of that characteristic that falls in one of the first three categories
5. The characteristic does not have high survival value

*Source*: Adapted from Fishbein, H. (1976). Evolution development and children's learning (p. 8). Pacific Palisades, CA: Goodyear Publishing Co. Adapted by Moffatt, A. (1993). Introduction. In A. Moffitt, M. Kramer, & R. Hoffmann (Eds.), The functions of dreaming (pp. 2–3). Albany, NY: SUNY Press.

neurochemistry, and electrophysiology. During animal sleep states physiologically similar to the dreaming associated states of humans, it is likely that some form of dreaming mentation takes place. Unfortunately, animals do not have the capacity to communicate content or to even report whether such "dreaming" is occurring. Dreams as experienced by animals may very well be like the thoughts of Wittgenstein's lion (opening chapter quote). They are likely to be radically unlike the dreams experienced by humans.

Animal dreaming fares poorly when comparatively assessed using human-based dreaming definition criteria (Table 3.1). Animal dreams meet full Axis-1 criteria (dreams occur during wake or sleep). But due to the lack of any dream report, such dreams have no reporting criteria (Axis 2) except observed movements. Axis 3 (dream content) must be inferred by an outside observer as based on the movements and sounds that take place while the animal is sleeping, or from areas of brain activation noted during REM sleep. It is possible that animal dreaming differs from human dreaming in being more likely to produce movements and vocalizations during sleep. But as noted, such movements are not typically associated with human dreaming except for those rare individuals with the diagnosis of RBD.

Dreams can function in both humans and animals in the processes of threat rehearsal and emotional processing. Humans as a species have incorporated the process of dreaming into the processes of creativity and innovation. This form of cognitive processing may be species-specific, and there is little or no evidence that such a use for dreaming has developed in other species. Dream-associated phenomena are compared between humans, other animals, and machines in Table 3.3. Based on definition criteria, it

**Table 3.3** A comparison of dream-associated epiphenomena between humans, other animals, and machines

| | Human | Animal | Machine |
|---|---|---|---|
| Neurologic (anatomic and physiologic framework) | Sleep stages (EEG) neuroanatomic activation | Sleep stages (EEG) and neuroanatomic activation | Possibility of artificially created network |
| Movements and sounds during sleep | Dream-associated only in infants and in some neurologic diseases | Sounds (barks and whimpers) and leg movements | — |
| Reports (recall) of mentation from sleep | Present from all sleep stages | — | Present during system (sleep) modes |
| Bizarre or hallucinatory content | Present based on definition from sleep onset, REM sleep, and deep sleep | — | Present based on definition |
| Dream effect on waking behaviors | Feedback on cognitive functioning, alternative outcomes, emotional processing, decision making, threat rehearsal, creativity | Feedback on cognitive functioning, emotional processing, threat rehearsal | Feedback on cognitive functioning, alternative result outcomes |

can be argued that humans share more dreaming characteristics with their artificial creations than they share with other animals.

## ANIMAL CONSCIOUSNESS—PRIMARY AND SECONDARY

Philosophical and neuroscientific approaches to consciousness, typically limit themselves to the phenomena that can be studied. Classification systems have been developed that divide animal consciousness into areas referred to as primary, secondary, and tertiary. Primary consciousness is the ability to integrate and respond to the special-sensory aspects of perception (auditory, visual, tactile, taste, olfactory) as well as the experience of pain and other body sensations (temperature and proprioception). Secondary conscious processes are those that cognitively integrate these perceptual and sensory inputs into thoughts, emotions, sense-of-self, learning, mental imagery, and orientation.[28] Executive-level (tertiary) conscious processes globally integrate aspects of primary and secondary consciousness. Tertiary-level functions include organization, planning, creativity, self-reflective awareness, execution of goal-directed behavior, flexibility of response to changing contingencies, volition, task persistence despite distraction, and dream incorporation into waking behavior.[29] It is such tertiary functions that allow humans to function and interact in their complex environment.

Many researchers into animal consciousness focus on its primary or secondary aspects. Very primitive animals and even some plants process and respond to perceptual information. This form of cognition, present in organisms without brains and even those without nuclei, is a form of primary consciousness. Researchers and theorists focused on primary aspects of consciousness can sometimes reach the conclusion that since almost everything in our environment responds to that environment, much of our surrounding environment is therefore alive and experiencing primary consciousness.[30]

More complex organisms are commissural, comprised of potentially independent constituents (cells) organized to work together as a larger mutually dependent organism. Almost all commissural animals demonstrate aspects of secondary consciousness: capacities for thought, emotion, learning, mental imagery, orientation in space, remembering, problem solving, rule and concept formation, and recognition.[31] Such cognitive capacities are species-specific, and accomplished by some species much more easily than by others.[32]

## TERTIARY ASPECTS OF ANIMAL CONSCIOUSNESS

Some animals experience and express the more complex tertiary levels of consciousness. There are animals that demonstrate cognitive capacities for learning, remembering, problem solving, rule and concept formation, perception, and recognition.[33] Darwin, among others, was impressed that animals have the clear capacity to express their emotions, suggesting that they have the capacity for "feeling."[34] Behaviors such as extreme reactions to the loss of a child or mate are expressed in many species. The apparent grieving and grave-site visitations by wild elephants and the collusive group expression and "singing" of cetaceans strongly suggest the presence in these animals of forms of executive/tertiary consciousness that are in some ways equivalent to our own. Yet, consciousness is a state both complicated and poorly defined. It has been difficult to find a way to study such behaviors, beyond their description, in creatures with whom we have only very limited communication. Most researchers and theorists restrict themselves from a methodological standpoint to studying testable, if limited, behavioral criteria such as attention, intention, and self-awareness that are the apparent tertiary levels of animal consciousness.

## ATTENTION

The most commonly studied tertiary aspect of consciousness is attention—a drawing of processing resources towards one particular object more than others. Attention is clearly an aspect of focused waking consciousness.[35] Our conceptual and implicit understanding of attention has changed somewhat since the topic was addressed in 1890 by William James:

> Everyone knows what attention is. It is the taking possession by the mind, in a clear and vivid form, of one out of what seem to be several simultaneously possible objects or trains of thought. Focalization, concentration of consciousness are of its essence. It implies withdrawal from some things in order to deal effectively with others.[36]

Today attention is considered to have at least three components: executive attention, alerting, and orienting. What James described as attention is now called "executive attention," the component of attention involved in focusing and narrowing the focus of attention. Alerting is a rapid response to perceptual and sense input, characterized in psychological testing by an increased error rate compared to executive attention. Orienting is the process of positioning and placement with reference to time and place.[37] Because some volitional control of the focus of awareness is possible, it is sometimes referred to as *attention/awareness*.

## INTENTION

Many philosophers approach the overall concept of consciousness by addressing the process of intention. The question of intention was a favorite topic for Socrates. Intentionality, coined as a term by Thomas Aquinas, is based on the Latin verb *intendo* (meaning to point at, aim at, or extend toward). In the 19th century Franz Bretano suggested that intentionality was the defining distinction characterizing mental phenomena, an irreducible feature of consciousness.[38] Friedrich Nietzsche once asked: "I notice something and seek a reason for it: this means originally: I seek attention in it, and above all someone who has intentions, a subject, a doer: every event a deed—formerly one saw intentions in all events, this is our oldest habit. Do animals possess it?"[39] Intention is clearly an aspect of tertiary consciousness. It is not unusual for humans to attribute intentionality to other humans and to animals, particularly to those other mammals who are their pets.[40]

## SELF-AWARENESS AND REFLEXIVE CONSCIOUSNESS (DEMASIO'S DOG)

*Self-awareness*, the awareness of being aware, has received considerable focus in animals.[31] The sense of self-awareness, based on the ability to recognize a mirror image as a representation of their own body, is a tertiary capability demonstrated by chimpanzees, orangutans, and gorillas that have been trained to use communicative gestures with human trainers.[32] Such a response pattern is often anecdotally described as present in some pets (cats and dogs). But experimentally it has only been demonstrated in elephants, dolphins, magpies, and some ants.[41]

It has been more difficult to empirically demonstrate that animals have the capacity for subjective experience—the capacity variously defined as reflexive consciousness and mind.[38] Behaviors such as emotional expression, and studies such as the mirror test suggest the possibility that some animals may have a "theory of mind"—the ability to logically think about their mental experiences as well as the behaviors of others.[33] In humans, dreams are self-referential and self-reflexive experiences, and viewed as such, are aspects of tertiary consciousness.[42] The incorporation of dreams into waking behaviors clearly involves executive/tertiary levels of conscious integration.[43] Antonio Damasio (1999) reached the conclusion that animals experience self-referential dreaming because their observed sleep-associated behavior includes emotional expressions that reflect feelings that they are experiencing in their dreams.[12] If this is true, such animals can be considered as quite special, demonstrating human-equivalent levels of tertiary reflexive consciousness while asleep.

## ANIMAL CONSCIOUSNESS—LIONS AND BATS

It seems clear that there are animals that share forms of consciousness with humans. The conscious states of animals are structured on a framework of biological systems that are very similar to those utilized by humans. And, because of this, our animal relatives surely have components of their conscious processing and dreaming that are similar to our own. Focused awake, default awake, and drowsiness, as well as some forms of sleep-associated mentation, are all states of consciousness that are behaviorally apparent in many mammals. Other conscious states are defined by cognition rather than observable behaviors. These states are more difficult to address in animals since they do not have the ability to communicate to us their reports of dreams or thought. We as humans have a clear tendency to anthropomorphize in ascribing human attributes to our animals, so that it seems quite obvious that my cat who keeps one eye open while luxuriating in the warmth of the sun, must clearly be meditating on the state of the universe.

The forms of animal consciousness, despite their similarities in biological framework to our own, are likely to be very unlike human forms. Animal perceptual and neurocognitive processing systems are markedly different from those utilized by humans. As the philosopher Tomas Nagel has queried, "What is it like to think like a bat?"[44] The dreams and thoughts of such a creature would be based on a waking world defined by ultrasonic sounds and their reflections, rather than by light and vision. Their structure of associative memory and emotions is likely to be even more different. Their consciousness of their-selves and their worlds must be at least as incomprehensible as the thoughts of a lion, and perhaps as difficult and strange as the dreams and consciousness of a machine.

# Notes

1. Wittgenstein, L. (1958). *Philosophical investigations* (p. 223). Oxford, UK: Blackwell. Another gnomic comment, but one which has extended itself into an entire area of philosophy that continues its development into the present day.
2. Aristotle (~350 B.C.) "The History of Animals." Barnes, J. (Ed.). (1984). *Complete works of Aristotle, volume 1: Revised Oxford translation*. Princeton, NJ: Princeton University Press.
3. Mallick, B. N., Pandi-Perumal, S. R., McCarley, R. W., & Morrison, A. R. (2011). *Rapid eye movement sleep: Regulation and function* (pp. 1−14). Cambridge, UK and New York: Cambridge University Press.
4. Solms, M. (1997). *The neuropsychology of dreams: A clinico-anatomical study*. Mahwah, NJ: Lawrence Erlbaum Associates; Solms, M., & Turnbull, O. (2002). *The brain and the inner world: An introduction to the neuroscience of subjective experience* (pp. 141−143). New York: Other Press. Professor Solms, more than any other, has had the authority and presented the logic in a fashion so that even those outside the dream field have finally come to the understanding that there is no clear indication that REM sleep has a special relationship with dreaming.
5. Verma, N., & Kushida, C. (2014). Restless legs and PLMD. In J. F. Pagel & S. R. Pandi-Perumal (Eds.), *Primary care sleep disorders: A practical guide* (2nd ed., pp. 339−344). New York: Springer Press.
6. Rechtschaffen, A., & Kales, A. (Eds.). (1968). *A manual of standardized terminology, techniques and scoring system for sleep stages of human subjects*. Los Angeles, CA: BI/BR. The classic scoring manual for sleep that defined the field has recently been replaced and "updated" by the American Academy of Sleep Medicine with a more dogmatic and less flexible version to be utilized in the technical scoring of sleep by sleep technicians.
7. Foulks, D. (1985). *Dreaming: A cognitive-psychological analysis*. Hillsdale, NJ: Lawrence Erlbaum Associates. A classic of dream science.
8. Valli, K., Frauscher, B., Gschliesser, V., Wolf, E., Falkerstetter, T., Schonwald, S., et al. (2011). Can observers link dream content to behaviors in rapid eye movement sleep behavior disorder? A cross-sectional experimental pilot study. *Journal of Sleep Research, 21*, 21−29. A group that continues to ask cogent questions of what we think that we understand about dreaming.
9. Gross, C. (1995). Aristotle on the brain. *The Neuroscientist, 1*(4), 245−250.
10. Coren, S. (2010). *Psychology today*. <https://www.psychologytoday.com/blog/canine-corner/201010/do-dogs-dream> Accessed 09.09.16. It is unclear how this individual became a specialist in animal dreaming.
11. Dement, W., & Vaughan, C. (2000). *The promise of sleep*. New York: Dell Trade Paperback. The history of the sleep science field by its founder.
12. Damasio, A. (1999). *The feeling of what happens: Body and emotion in the making of consciousness* (p. 100). New York: Harcourt Brace. A neurologist steps outside his field to develop theories of neuroconsciousness.
13. Google. (2014). *Google goes more Apple than ever in ad for rebranded mobile app*. Tech Culture. <www.cnet.com> Accessed 09.09.16.
14. Revonsuo, A., Tuominen, J., & Valli, K. (2015). The avatars in the machine: Dreaming as a simulation of social reality. In T. Metzinger & J. M. Windt (Eds.), *Open MIND*. Frankfurt am Main: MIND Group. Others looking at dreams outside the biological system.
15. Gould, S., & Lewontin, R. (1979). The spandrels of San Marco and the Panglossian paradigm: A critique of the adaptationist programme. *Proceedings of the Royal Society of London. Series B, 205*, 581−588.

16. Pagel, J. F. (2015). Treating nightmares: Sleep medicine and posttraumatic stress disorder. *Journal of Clinical Sleep Medicine*, *11*(1), 9—10. The politics of PTSD are almost as disturbing as the illness and its unaddressed effects.
17. Wynn, T., & Coolidge, F. L. (2012). *How to think like a Neandertal* (pp. 71—72). New York: Oxford University Press; Lewis-Williams, D., & Pearce, D. (2005). *Inside the Neolithic mind*. London: Thames and Hudson.
18. Barrett, D. (2001). *The committee of sleep: How artists, scientists and athletes use their dreams for creative problem solving*. New York: Crown/Random House.
19. Pagel, J. F., & Kwiatkowski, C. F. (2003). Creativity and dreaming: Correlation of reported dream incorporation into awake behavior with level and type of creative interest. *Creativity Research Journal*, *15*(2&3), 199—205.
20. Pagel, J. F. (2008). *The limits of dream: A scientific exploration of the mind/brain interface*. Oxford: Academic Press.
21. Pagel, J. F. (2014). *Dream science: Exploring the forms of consciousness*. Amsterdam and Boston, MA: Academic Press (Elsevier).
22. Fishbein, H. (1976). *Evolution development and children's learning* (p. 8). Pacific Palisades, CA: Goodyear Publishing Co. Adapted by Moffatt, A. (1993). Introduction. In A. Moffitt, M. Kramer, & R. Hoffmann (Eds.), *The functions of dreaming* (pp. 2—3). Albany, NY: SUNY Press.
23. Freud, S. (1953). The interpretation of dreams. In S. James (Ed.), *The standard editions of the complete psychological works of Sigmund Freud* (Vols. IV and V). London: Hogarth Press.
24. Pagel, J. F. (2011). REMS and dreaming: Historical perspectives. In B. N. Mallick, S. R. Pandi-Perumal, R. W. McCarley, & A. R. Morrison (Eds.), *Rapid eye movement sleep: Regulation and function* (pp. 1—14). Cambridge, UK and New York: Cambridge University Press.
25. Smith, C. (2010). Sleep states, memory processing and dreams. In J. F. Pagel (Ed.), *Dreaming and nightmares* (pp. 217—228). *Sleep Medicine Clinics*, *5*(2). Philadelphia, PA: Saunders/Elsevier. An excellent and even-handed review of sleep, dreams and memory.
26. Crick, F., & Mitchenson, G. (1983). The function of dream sleep. *Nature*, *304*, 111—114.
27. Hobson, J. A. (1996). *Consciousness* (p. 16). New York: Scientific American Library.
28. Roitblat, H. (1987). *Introduction to comparative cognition*. New York: Freeman. There is an entire field of animal consciousness that extends far beyond this overview presented from the machine perspective.
29. Shettleworth, S. (1972). Constraints on learning. In D. Lehrman, R. Hinde, & E. Shaw (Eds.), *Advances in the study of behavior*. New York: Academic Press.
30. Koch, C. (2013). Interviewer, Keim, B. (2013, November 14). A neuroscientist's radical theory of how networks become conscious. *Wired*.
31. Griffin, D. (2001). *Animal minds: Beyond cognition to consciousness* (pp. 23—25). Chicago, IL and London: University of Chicago Press. The forms of animal consciousness are even more diverse than human variants since almost all species exhibit multiple forms of consciousness.
32. Gorillas, L. (1994). Self-recognition and self-awareness. In S. Parker, R. Mitchell, & M. Boccia (Eds.), *Self-awareness in animals and humans: Developmental perspectives*. New York: Cambridge University Press.
33. Tomascello, M., & Call, J. (1997). *Primate cognition*. New York: Oxford University Press.
34. Darwin, C. (1872/2007). *The expression of the emotions in men and animals*. Mineola, NY: Dover Publications, Inc. The study of emotional expression is one of the oldest fields of cognitive psychology.

35. Demasio, A. (2010). *Self comes to mind: Constructing the conscious brain* (p. 203). New York: Pantheon Books.
36. James, W. (1890) The Principles of Psychology. New York: Henry Holt. Vol 1. pp. 403−4. From the same era as Darwin and Nietzsche—very smart and perceptive views of human behavioral expression.
37. Posner, M. (1994). Attention: The mechanisms of consciousness. *Proceedings of the National Academy of Sciences*, *91*, 7398−7403.
38. Gregory, R. (1987). *The Oxford companion to the mind*. New York: Oxford University Press.
39. Nietzsche, F. (1966). *Beyond good and evil* (W. Kaufmann, Trans.). New York: Vintage Books (Original work published 1886).
40. Pagels, H. R. (1988). *The dreams of reason: The computer and the rise of the sciences of complexity* (pp. 230−232). New York: Bantam Books. Another climber.
41. *List of animals that have passed the mirror test-animal cognition.* <www.animalcognition.org/2015/04/> Accessed 08.11.16.
42. Suzuki, H., Uchiyama, M., Tagaya, H., Ozaki, A., Kuriyama, K., Aritake, S., et al. (2004). Dreaming during non-rapid eye movement sleep in the absence of prior rapid eye movement sleep. *Sleep*, *27*(8), 1486−1490.
43. Pagel, J., & Vann, B. (1997). Cognitive organization of dream mentation: Evidence for correlation with memory processing systems. *ASDA Abstracts*.
44. Nagel, T. (1974). What is it like to be a bat? *The Philosophical Review*, *83*(4), 435−450. Today's response and extension of Wittgenstein.

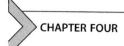

# CHAPTER FOUR

# Testing for Machine Consciousness

*We have long been accustomed to machinery which easily outperforms us in physical ways. That causes us no distress. On the contrary, we are only too pleased to have devices which regularly propel us at great speeds across the ground—a good five times as fast as the swiftest human athlete…We are even more delighted to have machines that can enable us physically to do things we have never been able to do before: they can lift us into the sky and deposit us at the other side of an ocean in a manner of hours. These achievements do not worry our pride. But to be able to think—that has been a very human prerogative. It has after all, been that ability to think which, when translated to physical terms, has enabled us to transcend our human limitations, and which has seemed to set us above our fellow creatures in achievement. If machines can one day excel us in that one important quality in which we have believed ourselves to be superior, shall we not then have surrendered that unique superiority to our creations?*

**Penrose R. (1989) The Emperor's New Mind.** [1]

Thinking, intelligence, data integration, and attention are aspects of consciousness. At the very beginning of the modern computing era, it was already obvious that machine systems could surpass human capacities in summation, arithmetic calculation, and code breaking. It was apparent that these systems had the potential to eclipse human capabilities in other areas. In society and in science, there was an intense anthropomorphic response to this possibility, most often presented as the apparently unarguable assertion: machines cannot think. [2] Confronted with the obvious intelligence of reasoning machines and the negative human reaction, theorists attempted to develop tests for consciousness that could be applied in testing systems for artificial intelligence.

Alan Turing, often considered to be the father of the modern computer, developed his "Turing Test" in the attempt to determine whether computational systems had passed the threshold of becoming conscious.

*Machine Dreaming and Consciousness.*
DOI: http://dx.doi.org/10.1016/B978-0-12-803720-1.00004-9

The test was introduced in his 1950 paper "Computing Machinery and Intelligence."[3] That paper opens with the words: "I propose to consider the question, 'Can machines think?'" But due to the difficulty that he was confronted with in attempting to define "thinking," Turing replaced that question by another that he believed could actually be answered: he asked whether an imaginable digital computer could imitate human responses so as to fool a human interpolator. Turing originally described the test as follows:

> It is played with three people, a man (A), a woman (B), and an interrogator (C), who may be of either sex. The interrogator stays in a room apart from the other two. The object of the game is for the interrogator to determine which of the two is the man and which is the woman. The interrogator is allowed to question A and B, but not as to physical characteristics, and is not allowed to hear their voices. The interrogator is allowed to experience or question only mental attributes. In the next step of the game, a machine is substituted for one of the humans, and the interrogator must differentiate the machine from the human.[4]

Systems including Mauldin's Julia (1944), Joseph Weizenbaum's ELIZA system (1966), and more recent chat-bots such as ALICE have demonstrated the capacity to imitate humans at least for a short period of time.[5] Colby, Hilf, Weber, and Kramer in 1972, demonstrated that their program PARRY in simulating behaviors similar to human paranoia patients, could not be distinguished from a similarly affected human by a physician judge.[6] Based in part on these results, the Turning test incorporated tighter constraints, including the requirements that such human imitation be of "normal" humans and maintained by the machine over time. As based on these criteria, no artificial system has yet been awarded the Loebner prize for fully meeting the criteria of passing the Turing Test.[7] If the Turing Test is a marker for human-equivalent consciousness, such consciousness is arguably within the capacity of intelligent machines. The Turing Test is basically an operational test for intelligent behavior, a test of the machine capacity for imitation. But even if the Turing Test is a good operational definition of intelligence, it may not indicate that a machine is conscious. Turing anticipated and attempted to dodge this line of criticism in his original paper, writing, "I do not wish to give the impression that I think there is no mystery about consciousness. There is, for instance, something of a paradox connected with any attempt to localize it. But I do not think these mysteries necessarily need to be solved before we can answer the question with which we are concerned in this paper."[3] Writing in

1950, Turing predicted that in about 50 years time, computers with a storage capacity of greater than $10^9$ would be able to play this imitation game so well that the average interrogator would not be able to have more than a 70% chance of making the right identification (man vs machine) after 5 min of questioning.[3] Today's machines are far more powerful, and since that prediction, it has been more than 50 years.

The philosopher John Searle derived the Chinese Room Test in form as based on the Turing Test:

> *Imagine that you carry out the steps in a program for answering questions in language you do not understand. I do not understand Chinese, so I imagine that I am locked in a room with a lot of boxes in Chinese symbols (the database), I get small bunches of Chinese symbols passed to me (questions in Chinese), and I look up in a rule book (the program) what I am supposed to do. I perform certain operations on the symbols in accordance with the rules (that is, I carry out the steps of the program) and give back small bunches of symbols (answers to questions) to those outside the room. I am the computer implementing a program for answering questions in Chinese, but all the same I do not understand a word of Chinese. And this is the point: if I do not understand Chinese solely on the basis of implementing a computer program for understanding Chinese, then neither does any other digital computer program solely on that basis, because no digital computer has anything I do not have.[8] (Fig. 4.1)*

This test argues that in order to have consciousness, a system must demonstrate more than the ability to manipulate formal symbols. A conscious system must also demonstrate mental and semantic content. Searle argues that external behavior cannot be used to determine if a machine is "actually" thinking or merely "simulating thinking." He has extended this argument to suggest that since computer programs can be designed to be syntactic (i.e., based on the grammatical structure of language) rather than semantics (i.e., the meaning of signs and symbols such as words), as for the man in the room who does not understand yet can still with direction manipulate the symbols of Chinese, the implementation of such a computer program will always prove insufficient in attaining basic aspects of both mind and consciousness.[9] Daniel Dennett has argued that this test of consciousness is confused and misdirected, "full of well conceived fallacies."[10] Colin McGinn, a leading light of the mysterium philosophers, suggests that such tests as the Chinese Room indicate that there is nothing to explain how the computational complexity of AI or the brain might give rise to consciousness.[11] David Chalmers, another philosopher of consciousness, in addressing the Chinese Room, concludes that,

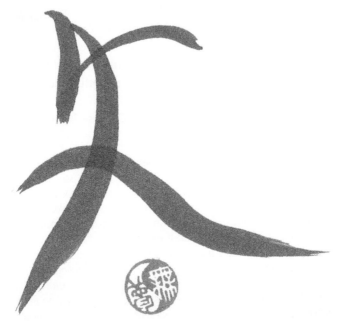

**Figure 4.1** Chinese for room.

"The outlook for machine consciousness is good in principle, if not in practice." From his perspective, the Chinese room is a test addressing the apparent limits of machine "intentionality" rather than a test addressing machine consciousness.[12]

Many papers, books, conferences, and organizations have debated the capacity of such tests to access for the presence or absence of consciousness.[13] But, as noted, consciousness is a poorly defined state. These tests have contributed more to the understanding of the state of consciousness and its definition than to the determination as to whether the animals or computer systems tested are actually displaying aspects of consciousness. What these tests for consciousness best describe is the capacity for any cognating system to meet the expected or required result criteria for the tests. Perhaps the capacity to satisfactorily meet test criteria will indicate as to whether a machine system has developed human-equivalent consciousness. The capacity attained is clearly dependent on the definition used. It remains unclear as to whether meeting such testing criteria would actually indicate that a system has attained consciousness.

## APPLIED TESTS

Beyond global testing, machine and animal capacity for consciousness can be approached based on the capacity of systems to parody, improve on, or extend conscious human capabilities. As Leibniz (1646–1716) once said "It is unworthy of excellent men to lose hours like slaves in the labor of calculation which could safely be relegated to anyone else if machines were used."[14] These labors may soon be over. Artificial intelligence as originally conceived was the capacity for an artificial system to simulate cognitive processes usually correlated with consciousness (Table 4.1).[15] AI systems have left many such definitions behind, with each definition seemingly disappearing at the point of applied intellectual analysis at which the AI system surpassed human capacity. Strong AI is now often viewed as an autonomous self-learning system with human–equivalent capacity and functioning.[11] Specific intelligence tests, primarily for assessing and defining human capacities, can be used in addressing the concept of intelligence in machines. These tests have proven societal value in assessing individual human capacities for applied intellectual analysis. These tests also address other aspects of consciousness including creativity, originality, self-awareness, and even autonomy. The ability to apprehend, understand, and guide actions requires that the individual taking the test have capacities for attention, developed intention, and goal-directed volition. Each of these aspects of consciousness can be addressed independently of the concept of intelligence. Each of these aspects of consciousness has been adopted and incorporated into specific epistemological fields of study.

Neuroscientists focus on attention, an aspect of consciousness that can be studied using real-time scanning and electrophysiologic monitoring systems. Intention is the domain of philosophers, with a long and argumentatively developed historic basis. Volition has become the focus for computer scientists intrigued by the possibility of consciousness in their artificial creations. Each of these aspects of consciousness is amenable to testing.

## INTELLIGENCE

Intelligence is a political term. It has been elastically applied in the past to assert that women, the brown races, and even machines, are not

**Table 4.1** Definitions of artificial intelligence

| | |
|---|---|
| [The automation of] activities that we associate with human thinking, activities such as decision-making, problem solving, learning ... | Bellman, R. (1978). *Artificial intelligence: Can computers think*. San Francisco, CA: Boyd & Frasier Pub. Co. |
| The study of mental faculties through the use of computational models. | Charniak, E., & McDermott, D. (1985). *Introduction to artificial intelligence*. London: Addison-Wesley. |
| The science of making machines do the sort of things that are done by human minds. | Gregory, R. (Ed.). (1987). *The Oxford companion to the mind* (p. 48). Oxford: Oxford University Press. |
| The attempt to find the primitive elements and logical relations in the subject (man or computer) that mirror the primitive objects and their relations that make up the world. | Dreyfus, H., & Dreyfus, S. (1988). Making a mind versus modeling the brain. In S. Graubard (Ed.), *The artificial intelligence debate* (p. 18). Cambridge, MA: MIT Press. |
| The art of creating machines that perform functions that require intelligence when performed by people. | Kurzweil, R. (1990). *The age of intelligent machines*. Cambridge, MA: MIT Press. |
| The study of the computations that make it possible to perceive, reason, and act. | Winston, P. (1992). *Artificial intelligence*. Pearson. Boston, MA: Addison-Wesley Longman Pub. Co. |
| The branch of computer science that is concerned with the automation of intelligent behavior. | Luger, G. (2001). *Artificial intelligence: Structures and strategies for complex problem solving*. New Delhi: Pearson Education. |
| A field of computer science that attempts to develop programs that will enable machines to display intelligent behavior. AI researchers still do not know how to create a program that matches human intelligence. No existing program can recall facts, solve problems, reason, learn, and process language with human facility. This lack of success has occurred not because computers are inferior to human brains, but because we do not yet know in sufficient detail how intelligence is organized in the brain. | Anderson, J. (2005). *Cognitive psychology and its implications* (6th ed., p. 2). New York: Worth Publishers. |

*(Continued)*

**Table 4.1** (Continued)

| | |
|---|---|
| Artificial Intelligence (strong) artefacts that have minds in the sense that we have minds. (Weak) artefacts which are able to implement certain functions which are held to be (weakly) constitutive of intelligence. Often used to sell white goods. | Carter, M. (2007). *Minds and computers.* Edinburgh: Edinburgh University Press. Glossary of Terms. |
| The holy grail of research into artificial learning and intelligence is, of course, to make an artificial mind smart enough to make another artificial mind smarter still. | Kelly, K. (2010). *What technology wants* (p. 259). New York: Viking. |
| Reproducing human consciousness. | Nicolelis, M. (2011). *Beyond boundaries* (p. 294). New York: Times Books. |
| As soon as it works, no one calls it AI anymore. | McCarthy, J.—attributed in Vardi, M. (2012). Artificial intelligence: Past and future. *Communications of the ASM, 55*(1), 5. |
| The Intelligence level of a human— Artificial general intelligence (AGI); An Intelligence level greater than a human—Artificial Superintelligence (ASI) | Barat, J. (2013). *Our final invention.* New York: Thomas Dunne Books. |
| AI is the field devoted to building artifacts capable of displaying, in controlled, well-understood environments, and over sustained periods of time, behaviors that we consider to be intelligent, or more generally, behaviors that we take to be at the heart of what it is to have a mind. | Arkoudas, K., & Bringsjord, S. (2014). Philosophic foundations. In K. Frankish & W. Ramsey (Eds.), *The Cambridge handbook of artificial intelligence* (p. 34). Cambridge: Cambridge University Press. |

and cannot become intelligent. The Turing Test and the Chinese Room Tests and their variants, and the game-playing tests of applied intellectual analysis are tests designed to assess intelligence (the power or act of understanding).[16] In most situations, intelligence is tested based on a subject's capacity to apprehend the interrelationships of presented facts in order to guide action towards a desired goal. Almost all of the tests designed to assess human intellectual capacity utilize this paradigm. Intelligence is, however, a difficult topic to address. It is most often defined by the tests used in its description. Turing suggested that unless there was something unique and magical about human intelligence, such a capacity should be attainable by computers. This is called the Church–Turing hypothesis: anything that can be computed by an algorithm or program can be computed by a Turing machine.[17]

AI game-playing systems have proved quite successful in applied games requiring intellectual analysis. These systems have proven superior to masters-level human competition for checkers, backgammon, jeopardy, scrabble, chess, bridge, go, and many other games.[7] Where these accomplishments were initially touted, now the surprising win of a human over a machine system is analyzed in detail, and seen as remarkable.[18] AI systems when applied to logical analysis have also been able to develop new approaches to the development of mathematical proofs.[16] The capacity clearly exists for AI systems to attain many human-level intelligence capabilities. It is very possible that in the near future, AI systems will eclipse human capacities in almost every applied, rule-defined test for "intelligence."

## ATTENTION

Attention (executive attention, alerting, and orienting) has proven amenable to modern techniques of experimental study. Real-time CNS scanning techniques including PET, MEG, and especially fMRI have been used to demonstrate that circumscribed areas of the brain are associated with specific areas of attentional focus. These studies have been used to identify specific CNS sites associated with topics of focus as diverse as pleasure, pain, and spiritual ecstasy.[19] A majority of the attentional sites identified by these modern scanning systems are not those postulated by earlier psychoanalytic, neuroscientific, and evolutionary theories of brain structure and function.

Most tests of intelligence have concentrated on the waking state of focused attention. Our educational system can be viewed as a program that trains us to establish and maintain the state of focused waking. Intelligence (IQ) tests of performance capacities during this state are remarkable in their capacity to predict school performance and later-life success in Western society.[20] Focused attention is the conscious state that is most likely to involve rational types of thought processing.[21] IQ tests assess the capacity to recall stored knowledge, what is sometimes called "crystallized intelligence," during a maintained state of focused waking. The ability to reason or solve problems using crystallized information is referred to as "fluid intelligence."[22] Some important attentional processes (e.g., where we move our eyes when we focus our attention) utilize cognitive processes that are nonconscious.[23] Attention is sensorially multifaceted, with each perceptual system (visual, auditory, tactile, and olfactory) controlled by a dedicated system for perceptual processing. The multiple processing systems for attention and behavioral expression are under central cognitive control. Parallel but separate systems executively control each sensorial network appropriately allocating competing demands for information processing.[24]

Much of the neuroscientific literature equates consciousness with this easier to study component of attention. This approach has been used to expand our understanding of the complexity of real-time attention correlates of neuroanatomy, electrophysiology, and brain function. Consciousness, however, includes much more than attention. Despite extensive training, most of us spend only a small portion of our waking existence in a state of focused attention. We spend a majority of waking time in a wide variety of "nonattentive" conscious states in which attention is de-emphasized, and other processes of thought, alertness, memory access, and time sense are prioritized.[25]

There has been a tendency for some experts to equate attention-based brain activation with consciousness. Brain sites have been identified that are activated by attention to diffuse concepts including spirituality, mathematics, and music.[19] Scanning data describing brain activation patterns during sleep have been used to "prove" that dogs dream about their waking experiences.[26] The Google interface can arrive at apparently logical conclusions, and authoritatively pronounce, "Yes. Dogs do Dream. And like humans they dream of their waking experience." From this anthropomorphic machine we are presented not with the results of logical analysis or peer-reviewed scientific study, but rather a dogmatic belief-based and anthropomorphic assertion as to what humans understand of dream consciousness. As noted from Internet reviews, the logic and proof of the underlying science matters less than that the style of presentation.[27] Perhaps we, as humans, need to believe that our dogs dream, and as well, need to use Google products.

## INTENTIONALITY

It is not uncommon for humans to attribute an intentional stance to machines and their programming.[28] We may complain that, "this damn program is blocking me!" or denote an alternative AI-based existence in which we "set up a meeting on the Internet." The intentional stance can, however, be used as an approach for assessing the presence or absence of consciousness in any system. The capacity for intention in any system, whether animal or machine, can be accessed by asking if an agents behavior is predictable or explicable based on that agent's intention.[11] Such an intentional system has several requirements: (1) an intentional system requires a capacity for thinking about something else outside the agent in consideration; and (2) the action or behavior is based upon an understanding of the circumstances involved. An intentional proposition can be diagramed based on components of attitude ($x$, $y$, and $z$) and the resultant propositions ($p$, $q$, and $r$): (e.g., $x$ believes that $p$; $y$ desires that $q$; $z$ wonders whether $r$). Neural maps of attention are hypothesized to comprise a resonance circuitry enabling us to be both self-aware and mindful of the intentions of others.[29]

From the machine perspective, an electronic construct of the intentional system already exists. Most computer programmers design their programming based on set goals for performance and function as required by the controller.[30] The controller that sets goals defines a required level of consciousness for that artificially constructed system. Today, computer language has become almost indispensible in accounting for concepts of intentionality in theories of mind.[31] Daniel Dennet, the modern philosopher who champions an intentional stance for approaching the question of consciousness, describes the computational process of intention as follows:

> The AI researcher starts with an intentionally characterized problem (e.g., how can I get a computer to understand questions of English?), breaks it down to sub-problems that are also intentionally characterized (e.g. how do I get the computer to recognize questions, distinguish subjects from predicates, ignore irrelevant parsings?) and then breaks these problems down still further until finally he reaches problems or task descriptions that are obviously mechanistic.[32]

Classically, the state of intentionality has often been considered as an all-or-none phenomenon. It seems clear, however, that intermediate levels of functional intentionality exist that are within the computational capacity of AI systems. Electronic detectors, scanners, filters, and inhibitors can be utilized to create AI correlates of intentionality.[33] Intentionality in the process of logical computation requires only a transducer (a device which takes information in one medium and translates it into another) and an effector (a device that can be directed by some signal in some medium to make something happen in another medium). Currently, almost all computer and AI systems intentionally store, use, and transform intention using electronic bits of information.[34]

The philosopher John Searle, creator of the Chinese Room Test, has expressed the view that intentionality is beyond the capacity of any non-biological system. He rests his argument on the problem of causality. He notes that intentionality as a biologic process is likely to be causally dependent and based on the response to biologic phenomena. He makes this argument as follows: "The point is that the brain's causal capacity to produce intentionality cannot consist in its instantiating of a computer program, since for any program you like it is possible for something to instantiate that program and still not have any mental states. Whatever it is that the brain does to produce intentionality, it cannot consist in instantiating a program since no program, by itself, is sufficient for intentionality."[35] It is Searle's assertion that behind the process of intention (the process of which can be artificially parodied) there is always causality. Causality, whether based on personal volition or belief, is a human/biologic construct. Causality and independent volition, at least today, seem to be beyond the capacity of constructed machines.

## VOLITION

Volition, what many view as the most important component of consciousness, can be defined as the ability to decide upon and initiate a course of action. Many of us use the concept of conscious *volition* as a central organizing principle.[36] In the human, in order for an experience to be considered voluntary, the experience must be accompanied by "conscious feeling of volition" or belief that one is acting and thinking deliberately and with personal choices in mind while taking into consideration possible options. An individual has alterative choices (regarding *what* to do, *when* to do it, or both) accompanied with a "feeling that it could have been otherwise." The volitionally acting individual is "consciously aware of the decision to act before the action is initiated...aware of decision and able to report it."[37] In experimental terms, volitional behavior is most often goal-oriented behavior (in terms of "set, strive for, and attain").[38] Volitional actions can be considered "free actions," philosophically defined as follows by Stace and Ayre:

A volitionally free action (X) is:

1. If desired an alterative action could have or would have been taken;
2. X was determined as a choice based on desires, beliefs, deliberation, and decision, and;
3. The agent was not coerced, compelled, or constrained in making this decision.[36]

Volition is often a component of problem solving, a dynamic that incorporates the processes of goal-orientation or striving toward achievement, accomplishment, and resolution. The volitional person or system exercises and experiences the feeling of personal choice, and the sense that things could be otherwise or different.[39] In human society and culture, volition is not always viewed as a positive attribute. Most religions include sects that emphasize the limitations and "sinful" nature of freewill, as opposed to the shared beliefs and concrete directions for behavior provided by the group. Politically, dictatorial and demagogic ideologues administer closed societies in which constituents accept having little or no choice as to options and behavior.

While both focused attention and intention are components of consciousness within the capacity of AI, volition is less clearly within the machine capacity. Strong AI is the concept of a system with the ability not only to operate autonomously within a predefined area of application, but to be completely autonomous within any general field of application. Such a system must have domain-independent skills necessary for acquiring a wide range of domain-specific knowledge. To reach this goal, a system must be capable of defining its own rules towards its own development. Only a "self-conscious" system is capable of (re)adjusting its own frame of reference and tuning its own rules (programming). For an AI system this potential is referred to as coherent extrapolated volition (CEV). CEV is what many computer scientists view as the machine equivalent to volitional human consciousness — the ability to "rise above programming."[40] To this point, there is little if any test-based evidence that AI systems have the capacity for CEV.

## SELF-AWARENESS

At some level, every independent organism is self-aware, living in the realization that it exists, requires nourishment, and perpetuation into the next generation independent of other creatures. For higher organisms, this distinction between what is inside and outside oneself is an inherent component marking the development of independent consciousness.[41] The development of self-awareness requires that an organism or system assume a privileged position, an inner life, from which that organism functions as a coherent whole. Dennett joins computer scientists and many sci-fi authors in arguing that it is this property of awareness-of-being-aware that would mark the capacity of an AI system to transcend programming.[42]

## AUTONOMOUS ENTITIES (STRONG AI)

The philosopher David Chalmers suggests that these components of consciousness (intelligence, attention, intention, volition, and self-awareness) are the "easy problems." These specific aspects of consciousness are easier to approach, characterize, and test for. This is as opposed to what he describes as the "hard problem" of consciousness: Why does the awareness of sensory information exist at all and why is there a subjective component to experience?[12] From the AI perspective, this difference is the difference been the concept of weak artificial consciousness (the capacity for a system that can simulate consciousness or cognitive processes usually correlated with consciousness) and strong artificial consciousness (the creation of a conscious machine).[43] Weak forms of AI are clearly within the capacity of a variety of currently operating systems that have moved beyond tight pro-grammed controlling to include aspects of machine learning in which the systems are able to modify their behavior in order to fulfill defined targets. A strong artificial consciousness would be able to take the further step of having the capacity to modify not only how it does what it does, but also to modify what it does. Such a system is playfully described by Riccardo Manzotti as having a teleologically open architecture ("what?").[44] Another way of describing such a system is as an autonomous entity. In order to consider any system an autonomous entity it must not only be aware of and able to manipulate its environment, it must also be in pursuit of its own agenda and be able to affect what it senses in the future. If desired, it could be within the capacity of such a system to appear as human if that met the requirements of that system. Such an artificial conscious being could appear to be conscious. It would have the capacity to act and behave as if it were a conscious human being.[41]

## DREAMING AS CONSCIOUSNESS

John Searle points out, "What I mean by 'consciousness' can best be illustrated by examples. When I wake up from a dreamless sleep, I enter a state of consciousness, a state that continues so long as I am awake. When I go to sleep or am put under general anesthetic or die, my conscious states cease. If during sleep I have dreams, I become conscious...."[35] The conscious states occurring in wake, sleep, and on the borderline of waking are each different forms of consciousness. Each state has behavioral, phenomenological, and neuroscientific aspects that allow it to be defined and characterized.[45] In the attempt to understand consciousness, the existence of these diverse forms of consciousness indicates that consciousness is not a unitary, or all-encompassing, state restricted or defined by one pattern of phenomenology.

The tests that we use to assess consciousness are derived from our perspective and understanding of human consciousness. When these tests are applied to other animals or machines, there is a tendency to hold those systems to tighter and perhaps higher criteria. Volition, intention, focused thought, and logical patterns of cognition are not present in some states of human consciousness, particularly the various states of sleep in which we dream. Any test of consciousness applied to animal or machine should also be applied to alternative, discrete, and/or altered states of consciousness in humans. These states, while different from focused waking, are still clearly conscious. Most tests for consciousness address components and characteristics—the "easy problems" of consciousness. Or they address the associated biological framework as it exists in humans. It has been more difficult to design tests that address the "hard problem" of consciousness in order to determine whether a teleologically open system, an actual autonomous entity, has been created or might be created.

For the early Greeks, the role of the priest/philosopher was defined as the capacity to determine which dreams were "true" and which were false. In order to accomplish this differentiation, they were forced to develop a version of scientific method: they kept meticulous records, and using empiric logic, successful results were utilized and failures discarded. Human dreams are clearly versions of consciousness differing from waking consciousness by their isolation from perceptual input and conscious volitional control. Yet, a dream as defined by its functions and effects—its roles in cognitive feedback, self-analysis, self-understanding, alternative problem-solving, and creativity—is likely to only be within the capacity of a teleologically open system that has the capacity to determine its own autonomous actions and project its alternatives into its future. Only an autonomously functioning entity could have such dreams. An artificial conscious being acting and behaving as if it were a conscious human being, yet not having subjective experience or mind, could pretend to report dreaming, but such artificial dreams would likely differ in form, structure, and function from "true" dreams. Today, it is within our capacity as humans to determine the difference between true dreams and false. The capacity for an artificial system to truly dream may in actuality be a better test for hard consciousness, than any of the other tests for consciousness developed to this point.

## Notes

1. Penrose, R. (1989). *The emperor's new mind* (pp. 3—4). New York: Vintage Paperback Edition.
2. Feigenbaum, E., & MeCorduck, P. (1983). *The fifth generation-artificial intelligence and Japan's computer challenge to the world* (p. 33). Reading, MA: Addison-Wesley Publishing Co.
3. Turing, A. (October 1950). Computing machinery and intelligence. *Mind, LIX*(236), 433—460. doi:10.1093/mind/LIX.236.433; reprinted in Anderson, A. (Ed.). (1964). *Minds and machines* (p. 13). New York: Prentice Hall. In another era Turing would have been acknowledged as the English Einstein, but an era of homophobia and power manipulation he was cast out from society, eventually committing suicide. This great man, the putative father of our modern computer based world, was destroyed by his fellow humans.
4. Turing, A. (1952). Can automatic calculating machines be said to think? In B. J. Copeland (Ed.), *The essential Turing: The ideas that gave birth to the computer age.* Oxford: Oxford University Press.
5. Gaglio, S. (2007). Intelligent artificial systems. In A. Chelia & R. Manzotti (Eds.), *Artificial consciousness.* Charlottesville, VA: Imprint Academy.
6. Colby, K., Hilf, F., Weber, S., & Kraemer, H. (1972). Turing-like indistinguishability tests for the validation of a computer simulation of paranoid processes. *Artzficiul Intelligence, 3,* 199—222.

7. Barrat, J. (2013). *Our final invention: Artificial intelligence and the end of the human era* (pp. 66–67). New York: Thomas Dunne Books.

8. Searle, J. (1977). *The mystery of consciousness* (pp. 10–11). New York: A New York Review Book.

9. Searle, J. (1984). *Mind, brains and science.* Cambridge, MA: Harvard University Press.

10. McGinn, C. (1991). *The problem of consciousness.* Oxford: Blackwell; McGinn, C. (2004). *Mindsight: Image, dream, meaning.* Cambridge, MA: Harvard University Press. McGinn in adopting the perspective that aspects of consciousness are outside our human purview, has created the "Mysterium" branch of philosophy, suggesting the possibility that reaching beyond concrete logics, consciousness can be understood.

11. Dennett, D. (1996). *Kinds of minds* (p. 34). New York: Basic Books.

12. Chalmers, D. (1996). *The conscious mind* (pp. 322–323). New York: Oxford Press. Chambers has championed consciousness as a topic of scientific study.

13. Chalmers, D. (Co-chair). (2014)—Towards a Science of Consciousness-20th anniversary. University of Arizona Center for Consciousness Studies; Tonori, G., & Koch, C. (2011). Consciousness Redux: Testing for consciousness in machines. *Scientific American.* www.scientificamerican.com/.../testing-for-consciousness-in-mach.

14. Leibniz, (1646–1716) as quoted in Smith, D. E. (1929). *A source book in mathematics* (pp. 180–181). New York: McGraw-Hill.

15. Padhy, N. (2005). *Artificial intelligence and intelligent systems* (pp. 6–7). Oxford: Oxford University Press.

16. Bostrom, N. (2014). *Superintelligence: Paths, dangers, strategies* (pp. 5, 13, 14). Oxford: Oxford University Press.

17. Rabin, M. O. (2012). *Turing, Church, Gödel, Computability, complexity and randomization: A personal view.*

18. Wood, M. (2016). The concept of "cat face"—Paul Taylor on machine learning. *London Review of Books, 38*(16), 30–32. Conceptually, our understanding of modern AI systems is morphing so rapidly that information is more often available from news-blurbs and on the Internet, than from books and/or constrained and intermittently accessible scientific publications.

19. Schuster, L. (2007). fMRI maps anatomical origins of belief in God. *Psychiatric Times.* www.psychiatrictimes.com/mri/fmri-maps-anatomical-origins-belief-god    Accessed 09.11.16.

20. Sternberg, R. (1997). The concept of intelligence and its role in lifelong learning and success. *American Psychologist, 52*(10), 1030–1037.

21. Wolman, R., & Kozmova, M. (2007). Last night I had the strangest dream: Varieties of rational thought process in dream reports. *Consciousness and Cognition, 16*(4), 838–849. Once again, an attempt to study dreams leads to a reconsideration of the types of thought processes that might actual characterize our waking.

22. Catell, R. (1963). Theory of fluid and crystallized intelligence. *Journal of Educational Psychology, 54*, 1–22.

23. Shiffrin, R. (1997). Attention, automatism, and consciousness. In J. Cohen & J. Schooler (Eds.), *25th symposium on cognition: Scientific approaches of consciousness* (pp. 49–64). Hillsdale, NJ: Erlbaum.

24. Pasher, H. (1998). *The psychology of attention.* Cambridge, MA: MIT Press; Anderson, J. (2005). *Cognitive psychology and its implications* (6th ed.). New York: Worth Publishers.

25. Andrews-Hanna, J. (2011). The brain's default network and its adaptive role in internal mentation. *Neuroscientist, XX*, 1–20. The discovery of the default network, widely dispersed CNS areas that activate as well as deactivate in concert with particular types of brain function indicates not only that other forms of CNS processing exist, but also that for global states such as consciousness, sleep and dreaming, such

networks may be far more important than classic transmission line neuroanatomical systems.

26. Coren, S. (2010). Do dogs dream? Dogs dream like humans and about similar things. *Psychology Today*. https://www.psychologytoday.com/blog/canine-corner/201010/do-dogs-dream Accessed 09.09.16.

27. Google. (2014). Google goes more Apple than ever in ad for rebranded mobile app. Tech Culture. www.cnet.com Accessed 09.09.16.

28. Pagels, H. R. (1988). *The dreams of reason: The computer and the rise of the sciences of complexity* (pp. 230–232). New York: Bantam Books.

29. Siegel, D. (2007). *The mindful brain*. New York: W. W. Norton & Co.

30. Taylor, J. (2007). Through machine attention to machine consciousness. In A. Chella & R. Manzotti (Eds.), *Artificial consciousness* (pp. 21–47). Charlottesville, VA: Imprint Academic. This important collection marks attempts by computer scientists and engineers to address the concept of artificial consciousness.

31. Lycan, W. C. (1987). *Consciousness*. Cambridge, MA: MIT Press.

32. Dennett, D. C. (1978). *Brainstorms* (p. 80). Montgomery, VT: Bradford Books.

33. Dijksterhuis, A., & Aarts, H. (2010). Goals, attention and (un)consciousness. *Annual Review of Psychology, 61*, 467–490.

34. English & English (1958) cited in Farthing, G. W. (1992). *The psychology of consciousness* (pp. 38–39). Upper Saddle River, NJ: Prentice Hall.

35. Searle, J. (1980). Minds, brains and programs. *The Behavioral and Brain Sciences, 3*, 423.

36. Ayre, A. J. (1954). Freedom and necessity. In *Philosophical essays*. London: McMillian; Stace, W. T. (1952). *Religion and the modern mind*. New York: Lippincott/Harper and Row.

37. Kilroe, P. (2000). The dream as text, the dream as narrative. *Dreaming, 10.3*, 125–137.

38. Voss, P. (2002). Essentials of general intelligence: The direct path to AGI. In B. Goertzel & C. Pennachin (Eds.), *Artificial general intelligence* (509 p.). Berlin: Springer. http://www.adaptiveai.com/research/index.htm.

39. Norretranders, T. (1998). *The user illusion* (p. 322). New York: Viking Press.

40. Franklin, S., & Graesser, A. (1997). Is it an agent, or just a program? A taxonomy for autonomous agent. In J. Muller, M. Woodridge, & N. Jennings (Eds.), *Intelligent agents III: Agent theories, architectures and languages* (pp. 21–35). Berlin: Springer.

41. Tagliasco, V. (2007). Artificial consciousness: A technological discipline. In A. Chella & R. Manzotti (Eds.), *Artificial consciousness* (p. 21). Charlottesville, VA: Imprint Academic.

42. Why we need "Conscious Artificial Intelligence" Hans Peter Willems MIND| CONSTRUCT May 2012, last accessed 23.09.16. The current best statement of criteria required that might mark the development of consciousness in a machine system.

43. Holland, O. (Ed.). (2003). *Machine consciousness*. New York: Imprint Academic.

44. Manzotti, R. (2007). From artificial intelligence to artificial consciousness. In A. Chelia & R. Manzotti (Eds.), *Artifical consciousness*. Charlottesville, VA: Imprint Academic.

45. Pagel, J. F. (2014). *Dream science: Exploring the forms of consciousness*. Oxford: Academic Press (Elsevier).

# Machine Dream Equivalents

It is now possible to create artificial software and hardware constructs of the underlying biological structures in which dreaming and consciousness form. As a result, and sometimes as a side effect of this process, machines have increased their capacity to meet definition and logic-based criteria for attaining cognitive processing states equivalent to biologic states of dreaming and consciousness. In this section, each chapter addresses a different machine dream equivalent as based on definition, phenomenology, technology, and/or metaphor.

Chapter 5, Sleep Modes, addresses the process of machine sleep in both finite state machines (FSMs) and in networks such as the Worldwide Web (www). In Chapter 6, Neural Networks: The Hard and Software Logic, we consider both the hardware and software of neural net systems. Fuzzy logic is approached from the machine perspective. Chapter 7, Filmmaking: Creating Artificial Dreams at the Interface, is a discussion of the manner in which the computer interface is structured on the same components of dreaming that are utilized in the technical process of film-making in creating artificial dreams. Bidirectional human—computer interfaces are addressed in Chapter 8, The Cyborg at the Dream Interface, as are novel interface systems using nonsensory modalities to extend the capacities of the interface into cognitive systems utilized more often in sleep and dream states than in waking perceptual focused attention. The data analyses, results, and outcomes produced by such systems can be hallucinatory and imprecise, strangely structured, altered, askew, and as hard to remember as any biologically produced dream. The interpretation of such outcomes and processes are the focus of Chapter 9, Interpreting the AI Dream.

At this point in time, we have the technical capacity to artificially create almost anything that we can describe—even systems which we do not fully understand. We are in the process of creating artificial constructs of the large, multiscale, nonlinear, highly heterogeneous, and highly interactive CNS processing system. Chapter 10, Creating the Perfect Zombie, considers the zombie systems under current development that will be part of our near future. It addresses the structure and processing of these systems, as well as their prospective capacity for dreaming and consciousness.

This section is perforce, somewhat technical. In constructing this section, the authors attempt to incorporate logical and inductive perspectives that they have come to their machines, machines that appear at least on some levels to already have the capacity to dream.

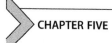

# CHAPTER FIVE

# Sleep Modes

*SLEEP (3) (suspend execution for interval)*
 *unsigned sleep (seconds)*
 *unsigned seconds.[1]*

One of the most profound realizations of our technical era has been that sleep, despite its lack of perceptual input, is an active state of cognitive processing. Before EEGs, and before real-time fMRI and PET scanning, sleep had most often been viewed as an off state of the body and brain. The only logical basis for inference otherwise was the reports of dreams on awakening.

Conceptually adapted, the biological state of sleep has been used to describe a series of "sleep modes" in electronic systems. The original purpose of the sleep mode was to offer a consciously controlled option for extending biologic sleep time. The offended human could reach out from bed and hit the "sleep" button on the alarm clock to shut down and delay the annoying alarm of waking. In this form of sleep mode with the electronic system turned off, sleep is a state of suspended execution with its limitations an extent defined by a timer (see initial quote).

Since their initial use (in mechanical alarm clocks), multiple forms of "sleep" analogues have been incorporated into electronic computer systems, denoted on the personal computer as low-power states (e.g., sleep and hibernate). In these states, the computer is not actively involved in the processing any data. These are suspended states in which the computer is preserved in either the system RAM or the system mass storage device. These sleep modes are power-saving states similar to when pause is pressed on a DVD player. In sleep modes almost all operative systems are turned off. Computer actions are stopped and open documents and applications put into memory. Full-power operation can be reassumed within a few seconds. Sleep, in a personal computer, is a low-power state in which the software state of the system memory is maintained. During sleep mode, your personal computer is not actively processing. The memory is not changed. The computer is in a quiescent state. An external stimulus can cause the "sleep" mode to be

*Machine Dreaming and Consciousness.*
DOI: http://dx.doi.org/10.1016/B978-0-12-803720-1.00005-0

exited. The source of this stimulus can be from either a timer, a user action, or such a programmed cue as a "wake on LAN magic packet."

Many currently utilized personal computers have an "Advanced Configuration and Power Interface" through which multiple designed global power states can be defined for a computer connected to a power source. These states vary from fully operational to connected but mechanically switched off. Four of these modes can be considered forms of global system sleep mode:

S1, Power On Suspend: CPU state and memory state are maintained, peripherals are powered off;

S2, Standby: CPU state and memory state are maintained;

S3, Suspend to RAM: Lower power Standby; CPU state and memory state are maintained "sleep";

S4, Suspend to disk: "hibernate."

S2 and S3 are for the most part identical and are often collectively called sleep.

In the Hibernate mode, open documents and running applications are saved to the hard disk while fully shutting down the computer. Once a computer is in Hibernate mode, it uses zero power. In Hibernate mode, a personal computer applies no power to either the system memory or the processor. Memory and processor states have been stored to the mass storage system to be restored at a later time. As in the sleep modes, the system may resume on timer, user action, or "wake on LAN." Once the computer is powered back on, it resumes where it left off. Some computers utilize Hybrid sleep modes that are a combination of the Sleep and Hibernate modes. These Hybrid modes put any open documents and applications in memory on the hard disk, and then put the computer into a low-power state, yet one that allows the user to quickly wake the computer and resume work. This Hybrid sleep mode is enabled by default in many systems. Hybrid Sleep mode is useful for desktop computers in case of a power outage. When power resumes, work can be restored from the hard disk, even if the RAM memory is not accessible.

## SLEEP IN FINITE STATE MACHINES

Computer processing can be broken into the categories of real-time and batch processing. In real-time processing, the processor performs calculations in response to changes of inputs, state, and time, and then generates output as a function of both the inputs and the state of the machine. The state of the machine changes as a function of the inputs and the defined present state. These systems are called Finite State Machines (FSM) the actions of which are described by:

$$state(t + 1) = Fs(state(t), inputs)$$
$$outputs = Fo(state(t), inputs)$$

For such machines there is a historical record of previous inputs and states implied by the present state. For a finite number of states there is a finite history. Such FSMs are the basic building block for computer software and hardware.

FSM microprocessors have become ubiquitous in appliances and other consumer products being marketed today. These processors usually have either a "low-power sleep mode," a "wait for interrupt" implementation, or a "wait for input change" mode that corresponds to an idle state for the machine. Fig. 5.1 is a flow chart for a simplistic "wait for input change" machine for opening and closing a chickenhouse door. This machine implements this program in two states, both of which are waiting for a change of the time of day from day to night or night to day; and then opening or closing the door. There are two basic types of FSM; Moore state machines in which the outputs are solely a function of the states and Mealy state machines where the outputs are a function of both the state and inputs. The act of closing the door is performed either by (Moore − state 'close door') or Mealy (state 'open door'

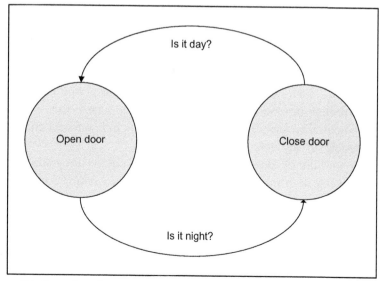

**Figure 5.1** Flow chart for a simplistic "wait for input change" FSM for opening and closing a chickenhouse door.

and 'is it night'). In both cases 'Is it day' and Is it night' act as the stimulus for inducing a transition to another state functioning as transition operators. An FSM typically utilizes parametric programming in which set numerical factors and operations define the conditions of operation. Such a system has no ability to deviate from the defined sequence or perform any other processing within this context. Programs can be utilized repeatedly during states of almost complete system shutdown. These programs are not dissimilar to those utilized to orient spaceships. During long-term periods of shut down, timed programs wake and compare sensor data to star maps, repetitively checking the maintenance of the ship's route and orientation in space.

FSMs as described in Fig. 5.1 are always in one of the two defined states—on or off. These systems are designed to implement the proscribed instructions in the order defined by the designer. For a delineated FSM, there is no programmed capability for lateral or apparently random processes to be initiated. FSMs may be implemented as either a hard entity in logic gates, a soft entity in software, or as a soft entity in a virtual machine incorporated within a computer software operating system. No matter the implementation, the operation is the same.

The difference between FSM machine sleep (an off state of no function) and biologic sleep (an on state with functioning that differs from waking) reflects a profound difference between machine and biologically based systems. Aristotle noted this difference early on. "What is [inanimate] is unaware, while what is [animate] is not unaware, of undergoing change."[2] Much later, in 1641, Descartes, using deductive logic, came to the conclusion that in humans, "A non-thinking, non-dreaming state is neither conscious nor alive."[3] Today, however, some neuroscientists argue that despite ongoing neural activity and reported dreams, the state of deep sleep is nonconsciousness.[4] There is little evidence supporting this perspective, beyond a relative decline in reported dream recall from the state.[5] Also, it is likely that in biological systems, as Descartes suggested, a fully off-state equivalent is not possible for any system that is actually alive.

FSMs are fully off during programmed sleep modes. Programs can be initiated during sleep mode as based on internally programmed or external cues. In order for these programs to operate, the system must be turned on. There is no evidence that any form of processing or data generation takes place in such a system while it is turned off. When off, FSMs do not possess the processing ability within their strictly defined states to support a logical analogue for the sleep-associated mentation correlate for human dreaming.

# SCREENSAVERS

*Opposite his chair was a stereovision tank disguised as an aquarium; he switched it on, guppies and tetras gave way to the face of the well-known Winchell Augustus Greaves. (Heinlein RA. (1961)* Stranger in a Strange Land*)[6] (Fig. 5.2)*

Virtual machines can operate within the framework of a physical machine(s). In an operating system, such an implementation allows one process thread to be "sleeping" while another process thread is fully active. A screensaver blanks the screen and fills it with moving images or patterns when the computer is otherwise not in use. Screensavers were initially designed to prevent phosphor burnout in computer monitors (hence the name), but are now used primarily to scrapbook photos and/or personalize the computer interaction. Screensavers are usually designed and coded using a variety of programming languages as well as graphics interfaces. Typically the authors of screensavers use the C or C + + programming languages, along with Graphics Device Interface (GDI), DirectX, or OpenGL, to craft their final products. Several Mac OS X screensavers are created and designed using the Quartz Extreme graphics layer. The screen-saver interfaces indirectly with the operating system producing a physical display screen overlaid with one or more graphic "scenes." The screensaver typically terminates after receiving a message from the operating system that a key has been pressed or the mouse has been moved.

The screensaver program is based on the execution of a sequence of stored instructions kept in the computer memory. The program follows an instruction cycle based on fetch, decode, and execute steps in its operation. These are typically simple programs that become functional during computer shutdown (off) periods. One increasingly popular application is for screensavers to activate a useful background task, such as a virus scan

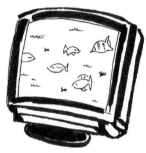

**Figure 5.2** The Heinlein screensaver.

or a distributed computing application (such as the SETI@home project). This allows applications to use FSM-based resources when the computer would be otherwise idle. When screensavers are implementing proscribed instructions in the order defined by the designer, the computer system is turned on, even though often operating independently of operator knowledge or control. Screenwriting system codes have proven susceptible to viral attacks and assaults allowing the computer to be co-opted by outside controllers when the screensaver mode is active.

Francis Crick, the Nobel Prize winning discover of DNA, partnered with neuroscientist Cristof Koch to develop what they called the "Astonishing Theory!" Today this theory is sometimes referred to as the "screensaver" theory of sleeping consciousness (dreaming).[7] Their astonishing theory postulates that what we experience as a dream is our conscious awareness of the unneeded excess of thoughts and perceptions from waking life that are being discarded during sleep. They propose that dreaming is a biologic form of computer system defragmentation and system cleaning, used in the CNS to dispose of and excrete nonpertinent perceptual data and experiential memories in order to improve waking function. Based on this theory, dreams are our conscious awareness of this nonconsciously active system. This approach to "dreaming" has been used by some respected neuroscientists to attribute and apply characteristics to the dream states. As based on this construct, dreams can be viewed as simpler, degraded cognitive processes than those that are involved in the processes of waking. Rather than having equivalence to waking forms of thought, it is suggested that dreams are composed of apparently meaningless and unneeded mental effluent that needed to be discarded to optimize CNS function. Since this theory was first proposed, other neuroscientists have expanded this construct, theorizing that dreams are a simple form of nocturnal hallucination in which more complex forms of thought and cognitive integration are not possible.[8] It has been postulated that the amount of integrated information that any entity possesses corresponds to its level of consciousness, with the level of structural "complexity" measured as simultaneous integration and segregation of activity during the state. The higher the number of connections and the greater the extent of integration in a system, the higher the level of consciousness that can be attained by the system.[9,10] As based on the screensaver perspective of dreams as simplified cognitive processes occurring during sleep, outside of the potentially nonconscious state of dreamless sleep, dreams can be construed to be a cognitive state with the lowest complexity and therefore the lowest level of consciousness attainable to the human CNS.

The screensaver theory of dreaming is a form of reverse-anthropomorphism in which machine processing requirements are attributed to human biological processing systems. Such theories date back at least to Newton who viewed the human as acting in response to applied mechanics and forces.[11] More modern versions base the programming of human actions on inherited genetic coding. Such machine-based explanations, as applied to humans, have a long history of wide theoretical acceptance, even when there is minimal correlative evidence. It is less often that human biologic and mind-based constructs are theoretically considered and/or experimentally utilized in considering aspects of machine processing.

## EXPANDING SLEEP MODE

During computer sleep modes, more complex software systems can maintain histories of events and responses. The form and format of this saved history is accessible by and maintained by the processor. These data can be used in the future to form new responses and processing actions. This is machine learning—in which the machine can deviate from the machine sleep state or an idle state to an alternative machine-selected sequence of states. This infers that the machine must not be in a quiescent state or must be caused to exit the quiescent state intermittently to process data. This deviation occurs when the machine is in an active on-state. That on-state can be induced or determined by some random factor, noise, and/or historical processing. Machine learning is only loosely controlled by the operator and provides this ability for the machine to develop or apply associated memories and approaches that can potentially result in different or unexpected outcomes. In Chapter 6, Neural Networks: The Hard and Software Logic, this form of "machine-dreaming" will be addressed in detail.

## NETWORK SLEEP

Computer networks are built upon interconnected nodes comprised of FSMs. Most often, these FSMs are general-purpose programmable hardware systems such as personal computers (PCs) and smart phones. The Internet is an organized system comprised of such nodes in which packets of data (batches) are transferred throughout an interconnected multiplex network.

These systems are exceedingly complex, built of heterogeneously designed and maintained components that utilize different and sometimes apparently opaque and cytogenetically unique computer and programming languages at each level of network architecture (Fig. 5.3).

In order to exist and function in a complex, physical, and often unruly human developed and defined world, networks must be far more flexible and adaptive than the individual FSMs on which they are built: nodes can crash and later be rebooted; fibers are cut; lightning strikes; electrical interference and thermal noise corrupt bits of data; switches run out of buffer space; data arrival rates exceed capacity; viral attacks overwhelm servers; and during periods of overload, managing software can forward packets of data into oblivion.[12] Networks interconnect systems that are heterogeneous in scale, type, routing, and language. Errors that occur in the processes of encoding, framing, data compression format, access mediation, and error detection can lead to situations in which data delivery becomes unreliable. Detecting such errors is only one part of the problem. In order for data delivery to occur, each error must be somehow corrected. Data correction algorithms can be inserted at the application level of the OSI model, but not within the modeled layers of the system.

Multiple techniques are utilized to address system instability. These include resource application techniques such as redundancy checking, switching, and bridging, used in the attempt to avoid problems of hardware and data packet contention, as well as queuing and congestion control. Error detection requires feedback retransmission in the event of either negative acknowledgement or the lack of acknowledgement for any particular

| End host | | | End host |
|---|---|---|---|
| Application | | | Application |
| Presentation | | | Presentation |
| Session | | | Session |
| Transport | | | Transport |
| Network | Network | Network | Network |
| Data link | Data link | Data link | Data link |
| Physical | Physical | Physical | Physical |

**Figure 5.3** The Open Systems Interconnection (OCI) model can be used to partition telecommunication and computing systems into abstract layers without regard to underlying structure and technology.

data packet. Each technique, developed in order to control known problems of system instability, adds to the complexity of overall network design and application. Each added layer of control must incorporate and include previously developed hardware and software systems. With each added layer of applied top-down control, the system becomes more complex and even more opaque to controller and programmer understanding.

System instability is at its highest during periods of congestion and high data load. It fact, the overall "power" of an interconnected system can be considered to be based on the system's capacity for resource allocation as based on the formula:

$$\text{Power} = \frac{\text{Throughtput}}{\text{Delay}}$$

The overall objective is to maximize this ratio, and to avoid situations in which the system throughput of data goes to zero when the system crashes during periods of extremely heavy load (the far right of the curve in Fig. 5.4). When this occurs, the entire network can experience an unstable situation in which packets of information are lost. Such an event is called a congestion collapse.

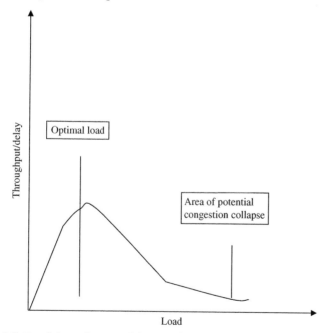

**Figure 5.4** Ratio of throughput to delay as a function of load (bell curve centered at optimal load with extension on the far right where increased load can lead to congestion collapse).

## BOTTLENECK ROUTERS

Any given node (source) may possess more than enough capacity to handle and convey a packet of information, but somewhere in the midst of the network, the batches of data will encounter a link being used by many different traffic sources that forms a congestion-based block that can interfere with the flow of information. In any given network, there is always a point at which such obstructions can occur. This point of congestion is often called a bottleneck router. There are several approaches that can be used to address bottlenecks that form during overload conditions. Route propagation protocols can be used so that data are rerouted and the specific bottleneck is avoided. The identified router can be replaced with one with more capacity. In each of these situations, however, the removal of one bottleneck in a complex system does little more than move the node site of congestion. Routers can be trained by using system maps that measure and then adjust for the shortest "hop" distance between source and destination. This approach can be used in the attempt to prevent the development of congestion bottlenecks occurring at different sites when the overall system is confronted with higher levels of load.

As with other machine processing concepts, the model of the bottleneck router has been applied to biologic systems. Consciousness itself has been proposed to be a form of bottleneck router. At the bottleneck of consciousness, only a small subset of biologic CNS activity is selected as accessible to conscious access.[13] The point at which consciousness develops is proposed to be the point of cognitive processing in the CNS at which data/memories are converted into self-generated internal representations of that data.[14] This point of access to consciousness becomes the major bottleneck affecting conscious processing. The attempt of various forms of CNS processing to surmount or alter the bottleneck router controlling consciousness could account in part for the development of the many forms of experienced consciousness—including the various forms of dreaming.

## FLOW CONGESTION AVOIDANCE

The attempt to alter or repair software or hardware bottlenecks in the system is a never-ending approach that can become somewhat like chasing a tail. Most attempts at reducing congestion attempt to effect and alter the allocation of available resources in order to avoid congested situations in which resources become scarce relative to demand. In any interconnected system involved in the conveyance of data packets, there is a continual pattern of increase and decrease in data congestion that exists throughout the lifetime of the connection. When data congestion is plotted over time, a typical sawtooth pattern results (Fig. 5.5).

During periods of high congestion, one approach that can be used to reduce data overload is to attempt to persuade some nodes in the network to decrease their use of the network. This can be attempted by using political or social approaches in which Internet access is limited—an approach often utilized by dictatorships and theocracies to limit assess to postscribed ideas considered antithetical to the rulers. But from the programming perspective, congestion is most often addressed within system context. Queuing mechanisms, incorporated delays and feedback are used in attempts to avoid the system timeouts and data dropouts that typically occur in highly congested interconnected systems. It should be noted that such programming applied during periods of high flow and congestion can increase requirements for data analysis and the complexity of applied programming, further slowing the rate of processing and contributing to degradation of service. Congestion control (the prevention of overall degradation of service when the demand for services exceeds system resources) has proven a difficult problem to address.

Changes in data flow also occur based on the patterns of human behavior. A sawtooth pattern of data flow occurs in response to the flux of data and available resources. It exists whether recorded on a second-to-second basis or when collected over a longer circadian 24-hr. cycle. This circadian variation in data flow takes place as a response to the changes in human

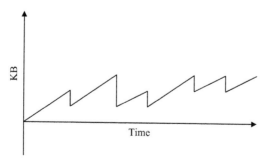

**Figure 5.5** Typical sawtooth pattern of data congestion plotted in kilobites (KB) versus time.

levels of data input and activity that reflect the timing of night/sleep cycles in high-population, high-technology segments of the globe. During these lower data-flow periods, system overload secondary to data congestion is less likely to occur. During these periods, the routing and data management resources available are more than sufficient to handle the lower levels of data flow. Interestingly, it is during these periods of "Internet sleep" that Internet functioning is able to adhere most closely to optimal performance.

# MACHINE SLEEP—SUMMARY

Sleep in FSMs is a mode in which the machine is actually "off" and without function. Screensaver modes are low-power alternative modes of machine functioning during which machine process and interactions can occur outside operator awareness and control. Screensaver modes are typically tightly controlled simple one-dimensional programs that function during computer shut down (off) periods. Dream equivalence has been proposed for screensaver activity in computer systems, functioning as a biologic form of defragmentation and system cleaning. Screensaver equivalent dreaming is of theoretically low complexity and integration. It has been suggested that the cognition associated with this process is limited and hallucinatory, constructed from degraded forms of mentation in the process of being eliminated from the system.[8] Screensaver theories of dreaming have been proposed as a potential outside marker for biological consciousness, equivalent perhaps to the dreaming-associated sleep state (stage 3) that is proposed to have reduced levels of cerebral integration.[9]

In AI systems, during machine learning the system can deviate from the machine sleep state to a sequence of states during which far more complex operations take place. For strong AI systems, these operations can include the integration of associated memories, decision-based feedback loops, and alternative or fuzzy logistics. During this form of AI sleep, potentially different or unexpected outcomes can occur that have even more similarity to dreaming in biologic systems. Such dream correlates will be discussed in later chapters.

In a system such as the Internet in which FSM (primarily PCs) systems serve as interconnected nodes within an extended system, a systemic form of sleep can occur. While individual nodes can drop out and turn off, the system as a whole is always maintained in a variable on-mode of interconnected data flow. From a systems perspective, the periods of low data flow in multiplex interconnected systems corresponding to human sleep periods can be viewed as periods of Internet sleep. As based on dream definition protocols (Chapter 1: Dreaming: The Human Perspective), the operations of cognitive processing that occur during these sleep periods meet all axis criteria. The data processing and results compiled during periods of Internet sleep can be considered as machine equivalents for dreaming. The possibility of Internet-based dreaming and consciousness will be discussed in far more detail (Chapter 14: Forms of Machine Dreaming).

For any individual system, the differences between machine sleep (an off state of no function) and biologic sleep (an on state with functioning that differs from waking consciousness) describes a profound difference between machine and biologically based systems. The absolute difference between sleep in machine and biologic systems is much less clear for independently operating and interconnected AI systems that utilize machine learning.

During systems-defined sleep, Internet systems demonstrably operate closer to optimal performance than during periods of high data flow and congestion (wake). During system sleep, exceedingly complex processing can occur. This complex processing is far more similar to what we now understand to be dream consciousness than the previously proposed computer science-based correlate for dreaming — degraded thoughts occurring during screensaver coupled defragmentation modes. Internet sleep-associated data processing has phenomenological similarities with human dreaming including highly complex, fluxing, always-on modes that include indeterminate and associative memory traces, and alternative, creative cognitive processing. Internet sleep-associated cognitive processing has much more in common with human dreaming than the cognition proposed to occur in association with screensaver modes. Interestingly, this data processing and its integration is at a more optimal level than that which occurs during data-congested states such as waking.

## Notes

1. Gehani, N. (1985). *Advanced C: Food for the educated palate* (p. 257). Rockville, MD: Computer Science Press.
2. Aristotle: Shute, C. (1941). *The psychology of Aristotle: An analysis of the living being* (pp. 115–121). New York: Columbia University Press, Morningside Heights.
3. Descartes, R. (1980). *Meditations on first philosophy* (D. Cress, Trans.). Indianapolis, IN: Hackett (Original work published 1641).
4. Tononi, G. (2008). Consciousness as integrated information: A provisional manifesto. *Biological Bulletin, 21*, 216–242.

5. Pagel, J. F. (2014). *Dream science: Exploring the forms of consciousness*. Oxford: Academic Press (Elsevier).
6. Heinlein, R. (1961). *Stranger in a strange land*. New York: Berkley. In the area of machine consciousness, the considerable contributions of astute and precognitive science-fiction writers such as Heinlein should not easily be dismissed.
7. Crick, F., & Koch, C. (1992). The problem of consciousness. *Scientific American, 267*, 152–159; Crick, F., & Koch, C. (1995). *The astonishing hypothesis: The scientific search for the soul*. New York: Scribner and Maxwell Macmillan International.
8. Hobson, A. (2000). Consciousness. New York: W. H. Freeman & Co. In order to protect activation-synthesis, the complexity, beauty, and significance of the dream had to be discarded.
9. Koch, C., & Tononi, G. (2008). Can machines be conscious? *IEEE Spectrum, 45*, 55–59.
10. Balduzzi, D., & Tononi, G. (2008). Integrated information in discrete dynamical systems: Motivation and theoretical framework, *PLoS Computational Biology, 4*(6), e1000091.
11. Newton, I. (1687/1999). *The Principia: Mathematical principles of natural philosophy*. Berkeley, CA: University of California Press.
12. Peterson, L., & Davie, B. (2000). *Computer networks: A systems approach* (2nd ed., pp. 304–305). San Francisco, CA: Morgan Kaufman Publishers. Written on a difficult topic for the outsider to the field—a beautifully structured and presented book.
13. Dehaene, S. (2014). *Consciousness and the brain: Deciphering how the brain codes our thoughts*. New York: Penguin.
14. Parasi, D. (2007). Mental robotics. In A. Chella & R. Manzotti (Eds.), *Artificial consciousness* (pp. 191–211). Charlottesville, VA: Imprint-Academic.

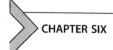

# CHAPTER SIX

# Neural Networks: The Hard and Software Logic

*The nervous system contains many circular paths, whose activity so regenerates the excitation of any participant neurone that reference to time past becomes indefinite, although it still implies that afferent activity has realized one of a certain class of configurations over time. Precise specification of these implications by means of recursive functions, and determination of those that can be embodied in the activity of nervous nets, completes the theory.*

**McCulloch and Pitts (1965) Embodiments of the Mind.[1]**

The human CNS provides each of us with the capacity for encoding information that describes the status of our external and internal universe. At its basis, in the biologic CNS, this encoding is a digital process, comprised of neurons that either fire or do not fire. Neural firing pattern encodes this information into set patterns of neuron interconnections, the vivacity dependent on the level and frequency of access. This trace is not dissimilar to the corresponding pattern of information process utilized in a digital computer—a series of on—off bits of data that compile data describing an external or internal process.

Mathematics, logic, and computer programs are built on digital on—off criteria. The nature of experience is, of course, not black and white. We live in a perceptual and philosophic world filled with colors, darkness, and shades of gray, in which it is rare for anything to be so clearly defined. Even in science, most problems are solved, not on a yes—no basis, but in relationship to the probability that a solution will apply a majority of the time. Statistical probability has become the proof of scientific experiment, and the basis for scientific logic and law.

For most humans the use and effects of probability on experience is rarely apparent. We gamble on the Kentucky Derby. And we invest in the local lottery using hunches and beliefs, despite the very high probability that we will lose. Our creations, our machines, however, are logically programmed

*Machine Dreaming and Consciousness.*
DOI: http://dx.doi.org/10.1016/B978-0-12-803720-1.00006-2
83

utilizing parametric logic and statistical probability in analyzing data to reach conclusions. Parametrically programmed machines often have difficulty ignoring the logic of their programming in order to function in the gambling, ill-defined and sometimes illogical human environment. Such systems require a directional override of logic in order to help us to invest in the lottery.

## FUZZY LOGIC

*So far as the laws of mathematics refer to reality, they are not certain. And so far as they are certain, they do not refer to reality.*
**Albert Einstein, Geometry and Experience.**[2]

Fuzzy logic is the concept of multivalence as applied to real numbers. Multivalence, applied to specific numbers within a range, is an extension of digital bivalence in which there are only two possible answers—yes or no, black or white, 0 or 1. For any question, the solution will include three or more options, introducing what can be an infinite spectrum of options rather than one of two extremes.[3] For a multivalued system based on fuzzy logic, the solution to any question is at least three-valued: true, false, or indeterminate. Immanuel Kant philosophized that our minds structure our perceptions, suggesting that our minds impose an infrastructure on our thinking by applying the principle of causality—the probable chance that an event will occur.[4] We use such approximations in determining potential causality—in our decision-making and in planning for our own futures. But, as noted by Einstein in the quote above, we rarely base our behavior on such a strictly defined yes or no mathematical reality. Multivalent logic fits better than parametric math with our human experience of reality. Multivalent approximation often typifies our waking human experience.

Set theory can be used to expand probability theory into the areas of dynamic vagueness generally referred to as fuzzy logic. It is helpful to refer back to the origins of the concept of fuzzy logic as developed by Lofti Zadeh in the early 1960s.

*There is a fairly wide gap between what might be regarded as "animate" systems theorists and "inanimate" system theorists at the present time. And it is not at all certain that this gap will be narrowed, much less closed in the near future. There are some who feel that this gap reflects the fundamental inadequacy of the conventional mathematics—the mathematics of precisely-defined points, functions, sets, probability measures, etc.—for coping with the analysis of biological systems, and that to deal effectively with such systems, we need a radically different kind of mathematics, the mathematics of fuzzy or cloudy quantities which are not describable in terms of probability distributions. Indeed the need for such mathematics is becoming increasingly apparent even in the realm of inanimate systems, for in most practical cases the a priori data as well as the criteria by which the performance of a man-made system is judged are far from being precisely defined or having accurately known probability distributions.[5]*

While many Western scientists and mathematicians have been slow to acknowledge the rationale behind fuzzy logic, the field of computer-science was quick to see the possibilities inherent in this approach. The applied results derived from using this approach have been profound. Fuzzy systems can model real-world dynamical systems changing over time. In many real-world situations, fuzzy systems perform better than more concretely designed parametric systems. Today they are utilized almost across the board in AI: in driving systems, appliances, routers, mass transport, etc. As Zadeh notes, "The closer one looks at a real world problem, the fuzzier becomes the solution."[6] Set rules of fuzzy logic such as data clustering and energy wells are now utilized in most AI learning protocols. Bart Kosko suggests that using fuzzy logic protocols an AI system when provided with enough data can learn to operate in any real-world dynamic.[3]

## ARTIFICIAL NEURAL NETWORKS

Neural logic computes results with real numbers, the numbers that we routinely use in arithmetic and counting, as opposed to "crisp" binary ones and zeros. Specialized hardware and software have been created to implement neural probabilistic truth/not-truth, or fire/don't fire logic. This multilevel approach to fuzzy logic can be used to measure variables as to the degree of a characteristic. Fuzzy state machines act on the multilevel inputs by a system of rules-based inference. Using a set of multiple variables and inputs acted on by multiple rules can produce multiple results with different probabilities. Since entry into and exit from any specific fuzzy state is probabilistic, there exists the case for autonomous creation of new states based on alternate state transition rules to a new set of solutions. Using historical data in a more mutable and adaptable form (sometimes called soft fuzzy logic) can allow the system to change rules based on previous data, and to then use that changed approach to create new states.[5]

Feedback is an intrinsic component of every physiologic system. A dynamic feedback system makes it possible for set in-points to be attained in response to changing conditions. For machine learning to be possible, feedback systems are required. The greater the number of feedback loops, the more precise the attainable response, particularly in fuzzy multivalent systems.[3] Feedback allows for the processing of scrambled, fragmented, and high-interference signals, and for the processing of data packets in which basic code data have been dropped or lost.

Artificial neural networks (AANs) can be used to perform probabilistic functions in either a hardware or software analogue. These systems are designed to operate in the same manner in which the neurons and synapses of the brain are theorized to operate. The architecture of neural connections can be described as a combinational feedforward network. In order to insert context, as well as to provide the possibility for feedback self-correction, some networks add a form of state feedback called back propagation. Once a feedback system is in place, the possibility of machine learning is present. In the process of machine learning, system behavior and processing are altered based on the degree of approximation achieved for any specified goal. In today's systems, the human programmer sets the specified goals. Applied system feedback, however, allows the AI system to develop alternative approaches to attaining the set goals.

The implementation of feedback systems can be on a real-time or a pseudo-real-time basis. Pseudo-real-time is a programmed process that provides a timeline-independent multiplexed environment in which to implement a neural and synaptic connection network. An artificially produced machine-style implementation of synapses and neurons (neural network) can be set up to operate in the present state, next state, or via synaptic weightings implemented as matrices. Computer programming languages and systems have been designed to facilitate the development of machine learning for artificial neural network systems. The Python programming language modules Theano, numpy, neurolab, and scipy provide a framework for these types of matrix operations. The Theano language provides an environment for performing symbolic operations on symbolic datasets to provide scalar results, useful when speed is essential.

Artificial neurons operate by summing inputs (s1,s2,s3) individually scaled by weight factors (w1,w2,w3) and processing that sum with a nonlinear activation function (af), most often approximating the logistic-function: $1/(1 + \exp(-x))$ which returns a real value in the range (0,1) (Fig. 6.1). Single artificial neurons can be envisioned as single combinatorial operators. More complex operations such as exclusive-or mappings require additional levels of neurons just as they require additional levels of crisp logic. Processes such as look-up-table logic can be used to implement multiple gates in one table by mapping all possible input combinations. Multiple-multiple levels of logic can be implemented in one table.

Supervised neural networks are programmed and trained to infer a set goal or solution based on sets of inputs and desired outputs. A solution is developed based on the result of a specific set of artificial neurons "firing" and being propagated to the output. From the programmer's perspective, there are typical problems that limit the capacities of such systems. These include noise (the incorporation of incorrect data points leading to a decline in performance), the need for invariance of a solution with respect to variance in multiple inputs, and the fact that these systems include a far smaller number of neural interconnections than an organic brain. These limitations of neural-network designed systems can produce multiple solutions from the same given set of inputs. Incomplete training sets are more often to lead to indecisive outputs.[7]

An example of an artificial neuron with training written in Python is presented in Table 6.1. Plots of training action are also presented. Note that not all inputs result in well-defined outputs. For this example, Fig. 6.2 summarizes the functionality of such a system. There are eight possible inputs, only seven of which result in definitive outputs, while only four are defined in training. The three definitive outputs resulting from untrained

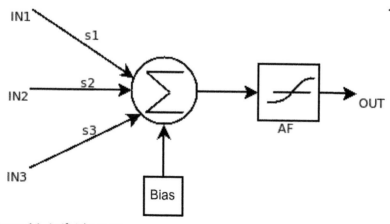

**Figure 6.1** Artificial neuron.

**Table 6.1** Simple neuron training and results

| Input vector | Trained output | Functional output |
|---|---|---|
| [0,0,0] | | [0.99995733] |
| [0,0,1] | | [5.91174766e-13] |
| [0,1,0] | | [0.50101207] |
| [0,1,1] | [0] | [2.53267443e-17] |
| [1,0,0] | [1] | [1.] |
| [1,0,1] | | [0.00673341] |
| [1,1,0] | [1] | [1.] |
| [1,1,1] | [0] | [2.90423911e-07] |

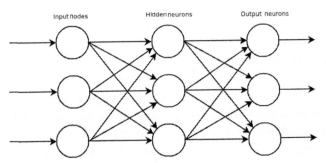

**Figure 6.2** Feedforward neural network.

input conditions can be envisioned as hallucinatory since the answers provided are hypothetical and nonapplicable to the real-world situation, yet are based on the same given set of data input. The nondeterministic output is indecisive and most often noninterpretable. Propagated to successive layers of neurons, the results of these nontrained inputs result in an additional level of unintended operation leading to unexpected results. The nondeterministic input condition [0,1,0], combined with noise on any of the inputs, will result in a randomness of that output as well.

Figs. 6.1 and 6.2 are neurolab neural networks that provide insight into multilayer neural networks. Their training and implications of undertraining are demonstrated. The corresponding console outputs for these examples show results for both crisp and real numbers.

Recurrent and reentrant neural networks (Fig. 6.3) implement connections from lower layers of neuron into upper layers of the network of neurons. Such a configuration can be used to provide a temporal/sequential dimension to neural network processing. From a control theory point of view, these connections can be envisioned as feedback. While feedback is most often a positive process, particularly in fuzzy

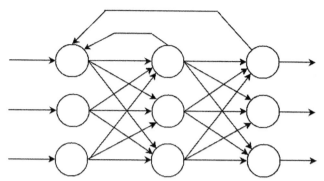

**Figure 6.3** Partially recurrent neural network connections.

processing systems, feedback loops can also contribute to indeterminate or hallucinatory results. Feedback allows for the possibility of creating multiple poles and zeros within the neural network solution space. Poles and zeros potentially allow the conditions of oscillation and latch-up, both unintended and undesirable, and both leading to incorrect or unusable solution results attained from the same data analysis.

ANNs are most often implemented and represented by matrices. For a $1 \times n$ matrix, N represents inputs, and I artificial neurons. Multiplied by a weight matrix for each neuron input, the summation becomes a sum of weighted outputs from all other neurons and inputs. An activation function is then used to calculate individual neuron outputs. For a state machine form with neurons and inputs represented by matrix N, weighting by matrix W, and outputs by O with an output definition matrix of U:

$$N(t+1) = af(N(t)W)$$
$$O(t+1) = af(N(t)U)$$

Neural networks can be "trained" by initializing the weight matrix W with either random values or with a set of suggested values and comparing the output O (I). Target values are established for a set of input values, and the desired output is derived based on individual neuron inputs. This value is calculated and W is iteratively adjusted to achieve the desired output O. As networks are made deeper and wider, and as the internal neurons are less defined and increasingly nonspecific, the ability to train becomes more difficult. Many repeated iterations are required for training a small network. Large networks require an exponentially greater number of training iterations and a complete set of training data to avoid undesirable operation results (such as identifying a cat as a dog). With the inclusion of temporal feedback to add time-based relevance to inputs, susceptibility to unintended operation becomes even more likely.

ANNs can clearly be taught. Learning takes place in a conceptually similar manner to the way that neural networks are trained to retain memories in the human CNS. Repeated and stronger interactions can be expressed and integrated based on probability factors, sometimes called signal weight. A network can be trained to assign weights to possible connections. Programmed rules can be set up establishing the parameters and limits for particular connections. An ANN can be trained in this manner to recognize errors, minimize rarely used synaptic paths, and adjust its synaptic weights accordingly. This process is utilized by current systems active in computer games, stock market analysis, and image identification in order to create systems that are inherently self-improving.[8]

Deep learning networks are neural networks that are extremely large in the number of implemented levels. Such networks require large computing resources, and a great deal of data for learning. These learning data must be presented as a defined data set that has conditions/paths goals, values, and positive/negative rewards programmed and identified. Given the instabilities previously described in implementing recursive networks, without extensive testing and complete definition of all possible input sequences including errant and noisy variants, unintended responses are commonly produced and often expected.

## DREAM-LIKE NEURAL NETWORK PROCESSING

ANNs are designed to incorporate neural-cell-based operations of overall on–off processing, multiple connections, multiple levels, and dynamic feedback taking place in temporal sequence or in artificial psuedo-time spaces. These processes include the associated processes of associative, multilevel memory, and cognitive feedback. For many individuals, dreaming functions in providing feedback insight into CNS cognitive function, particularly the functioning that occurs during sleep. Neural network processing, in adopting the dream-like processes of cognitive feedback and multi-level associative memory, is an attempt to parody biologic processes of dreaming.

Neural network feedback is, however, far more specific in its attempt to control discrete data points. Systems as currently designed include a much smaller number of artificial neurons than biologic systems. Attained levels of complexity are therefore quite low. However, as noted, even at levels of low complexity in tightly supervised systems using multiple levels of neural feedback, discrete and limited data analysis is difficult to train and control. Incomplete training becomes a significant problem if it leads to dysfunction in AI controlled systems such as motor vehicles.

AI systems also differ from biologic systems in that they are designed and structured around the attempt to reach set goals. Computer programmers and engineers, like Leibnitz, tend to consider the role of AI systems as applied calculators controlling a series of mechanical operations to achieve desired outcomes (goals). Goal setting is less characteristic of dreaming, though it is an important part of the process called dream incubation. Incubation is a traditional and time-honored use of dreaming in which the individual goes to sleep considering a problem that is being confronted during waking.[9] Some individuals tie this process together with the attempt to achieve control of that decision-making process (lucidity) within the dream state. Such goal-oriented dreams have been reported by artists, filmmakers, musicians, scientists, and particularly writers to produce useful and often creative results.[10] But most dreams, even most creatively useful dreams, do not incorporate set goals and do not reflect goal-directed behavior.

Machines keep a record of their experience, including a history of low-level instruction execution and correlated inputs/outputs at the highest levels. This history may or may not be retained. When utilized in soft fuzzy logic systems or in trained AI, this history can provide a baseline for producing new and potentially creative outcomes from even tightly constrained data analysis.

AI machine experience and training define the AI machine response. Neural network-based AI systems can only respond definitively to the stimuli to which they have been trained. The combinations of real number stimuli, noise, and partial or incomplete training make AI machine dysfunction more probable as artificial neural density increases. Neural network-designed processing can produce a significant proportion of outcomes that can be considered as indeterminate or hallucinatory. Biologic dreams are often indeterminate and are also at times hallucinatory, particularly at sleep onset, occurring just after the initiation of sleep. Biologic dreams, particularly nightmares, have the characteristic of seeming to be real, and viewed as such, they can be considered hallucinatory, providing an alternative and apparently real version of reality. Approximately three of the eight results obtained from simple neural network processing are indeterminate or hallucinatory. Such obtained results are often considered as evidence for machine dysfunction, hypothetical and nonapplicable to the real-world situation.

A data analysis conducted using fuzzy logic systems, AI, and neural networks, even an analysis based on set and controlled goals, is far more likely to produce unexpected results than a system based on parametric and tightly controlled logic. Such results are often outside the box, indeterminate, and/or hallucinatory. These results, rather than marking machine dysfunction, mark the level of complexity and flexibility of the system. In order to interact with interactive systems that often operate outside logical constraints (humans), it may be important to incorporate and include such alterative and apparently nonlogical outcomes. Is it anthropomorphism to consider, and perhaps describe, such results as machine dreams?

## Notes

1. McCulloch, W., & Pitts, W. (1965). A logical calculus of the ideals immanent in nervous activity. In W. McCulloch (Ed.), *Embodiments of the mind* (p. 21). Cambridge, MA: MIT Press. One of the classic papers in the field.
2. Einstein, A. (1983). Geometry and experience. In *Sidelights on relativity* (G. B. Jeffery & W. Perrett, Trans.). New York: Dover Press and E. P. Dutton (Original work published 1922).
3. Kosko, B. (1993). *Fuzzy thinking: The new science of fuzzy logic* (p. 19). New York: Hyperion.
4. Kant, I. (1781/1996). *Critique of pure reason* (W. Pluhar, Trans.). Indianapolis, IN: Hackett. From an era when pure reason could be considered as apparent in the human species.
5. Zadeh, L. (1962). From circuit theory to system theory. *Proceedings of the IRE, 50,* 856–865.
6. Zadeh, L. (1987). Advances in Fuzzy Mathematics and Engineering. In L. Zadeh, R. Yager, S. Ovchinnikov, R. Tong, & H. Nguyen (Eds.), *Fuzzy sets and applications: Selected papers*. New York: Wiley.
7. Gillies, D. (1996). *Artificial intelligence and scientific method*. Oxford: Oxford University Press.
8. Barrat, J. (2013). *Our final invention: Artificial intelligence and the end of the human era* (pp. 214–215). New York: Thomas Dunne Books.
9. Delaney, G. (1979). *Living your dreams*. San Francisco, CA: Harper Books. Gayle is still living her dreams in Los Angeles as dream interpreter to the stars.
10. Pagel, J. F., & Kwiatkowski, C. F. (2003). Creativity and dreaming: Correlation of reported dream incorporation into awake behavior with level and type of creative interest. *Creativity Research Journal, 15*(2&3), 199–205.

This chapter and the last are based primarily on the insights of Philip Kirshtein, the computer scientist that has partnered in this project. As he notes, he is an actual computer scientist, someone with more patents than papers, and someone who based on his work was able to retire from full-time work at an early age in order to work on such projects as his computer-operated chickenhouse door.

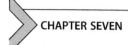

CHAPTER SEVEN

# Filmmaking: Creating Artificial Dreams at the Interface

*I propose simply to follow the suggestion that we should picture the instrument which carries out our mental functions as resembling a microscope or photographic apparatus, or something of the kind. On that basis, psychical locality will correspond to a point outside the apparatus at which one of the preliminary stages of an image comes into being. In the microscope and telescope, as we know, these occur in part at ideal points, regions in which no tangible components of the apparatus is situated . . .. Accordingly, we will picture the mental apparatus as a compound instrument, to the components of which we will give the name "agencies," or (for the sake of greater clarity) "systems." It is to be anticipated, in the next place, that these systems may perhaps stand in a regular spatial relation to one another, in the same kind of way in which the various systems of lens in a telescope are arranged one behind the other.*

**Sigmund Freud (1914).[1]**

At the very start of the 20th century, the Luminare brothers created a series titled and numbered as *Dreams*, foggy and jerky, black and white moving pictures that somehow resembled dream imagery more than waking perception.[2] Even then, film was seen as an attempt at creating artificial dreams. Cinematographers discovered that they could fool the "eye as camera" into perceiving a continuous moving picture with three-dimensional characteristics of depth and foreground by projecting a series of still two-dimensional images at a speed of 16—24 frames/s. At this frame-rate, the periodic repetition of projected pictures dissolves perceptually into a continuity, producing the mechanistic basis for the motion picture. This projection of images at a fixed rate creates a subordination of time to movement with the present a point moving continuously from the past into the future. The continuous projection of images establishes disconnection with objective reality for the viewer producing an alternative reality outside the chronological reality of our external (nonfilm-watching) lives.[3] In today's world, filmmaking is a

*Machine Dreaming and Consciousness.*
DOI: http://dx.doi.org/10.1016/B978-0-12-803720-1.00007-4

collaborative, technically complex process that requires a wide spectrum of knowledge. This can include an awareness of previously utilized approaches and techniques, a background in visual photography and cinematography, an understanding of visual science, as well as a creative approach to narrative and the process of story. Much of what we understand about the processing of visual information has come from attempting to understand the techniques used in filmmaking, techniques that fool us into believing that we are seeing something that we are not.[4] Vision is replete with illusions, both physical and psychological, as well as visual phenomena such as ambiguities (visual projections that occasionally match object reality), paradoxes (those that cannot be matched or measured as objects), and fictions (that have no objective counterparts).[4] Neuroscientists study the techniques of film in their attempts to understand the cognitive processing utilized for sensory vision as well as for mental imagery. Psychoanalysists and psychiatrists have used filmmaking processes as models in developing theories that might explain the basic structure of mental dynamics (see the initial Freud quote on psychical apparatus theory).

Cinematic language has provided a better handle for describing dreams than the sciences of linguistics, optics, electrophysiology, neurology, or the other philosophies. Beyond Freud, a short list of dream-adopted film terminology includes eye-as-camera, projection, point-of-view, crossing the line, the subordination of time to motion, and flashback. Films have the capacity to create an almost complete cognitive experience outside the viewer's control. They affect the memory systems, visual imagery, and emotions of the viewer. You find yourself remembering moments of a film, trying to find your way back to the mood and associations associated with a particular moment, tapping into emotionally competent stimuli that lead you down personal storypaths much different from those planned by the filmmaker. Films can provoke both nightmares and ecstasy—extreme emotions such as those experienced by the dreamer faced with his own creation.[5] As in dreams, certain moments of films viewed decades ago can be as vivid as moments of childhood, treasured moments that serve as a baseline comparison to waking experience.[6] The filmmaker incorporates the audience into an alternate reality, that, like dreaming, is sometimes better understood after reflection and integration by the viewer—an independently conscious process sharing characteristics with dream interpretation. Today Freudian- and post-Freudian-based film interpretation and theory form the "orthodoxy" of cinema study.

In order to create artificial dreams, the filmmaker (whether human or AI) must have the capacity to artificially approximate the biologic processes of dreaming. Dreams are structured primarily with visual images, associative memories, and emotions. It is very rare for a dream to not have these components. We take stored perceptual information and neurologically integrate our stores of memories and emotions into a representation of the external universe that we can interact with and cognitively understand. The filmmaker creates artificial correlates of these biological processes, integrating stored associated memories with emotions. But most of all, as in a dream, a film emphasizes the visual aspects of narrative story.

## THE VISUAL IMAGERY OF DREAM

When we are interacting with the exterior world or attempting to create representations of that world, we utilize continuous, explicit, and accessible perceptual input in order to describe the objects, the relationships between shapes, color, texture, and the spatial relationships between each point in the visual field. Waking visual processing is driven primarily by this sensory input. Dreaming, however, takes place during sleep, a conscious state of perceptual isolation. The only visual representations available are those stored in memory.[7] Techniques can be used to manipulate and fool the visual system at three different levels: at the sensory organ (the eye); in the visual neural processing systems; and at the levels of proposition and cognitive interpretation.

## THE SENSOR

The visuospatial system of our sensor (the eye) is responsive to a wide variety of stimuli ranging from color, to brightness, darkness, orientation, and motion.[8] The constraints of visual optics and the formation of images in the eye produce a portrayal of space and depth to the viewer—the eye as camera. This complex organ has the capacity to approximate at least some of the components of consciousness.[9] During sleep, eye movements occur most often during REMS and sleep onset, the sleep stages that are most likely to include reported dreams. The subordination of time to movement, the present as a point moving continuously from the past into the future, and the ability to perceive changes in chronologic time require an available physiologic marker. In waking visual perception, this marker is the physiological time lag required for the transmission of sensory information from the eye to the neural areas of cognitive processing. Our perspective of change in chronological time, as well as our requirements for sensing motion from projected still images, is based on the set limits of this physiological marker. In dreams, eye movements can function in providing a time-based marker by producing a neural time lag similar to that active during waking visual perception. Eye movements have the capacity to function as the sprocket in the projector, marking time and adding the fourth dimension to dreaming.[10]

## THE NEUROLOGICAL PROCESSING OF IMAGERY

Vision requires the largest area of the neuroanatomic CNS of any cognitive function. In the monkey, there are at least 32 discrete areas of the cerebral cortex that respond directly to selective visual input.[7] Vision processing is primarily a neuroanatomically defined process, so that the visual system is particularly available to the advances of modern scanning technology. Two major sophisticated cortical systems and one subcortical visual buffering system integrate visual content with memory systems and conscious activity.[11,12] One cortical system is organized based on point-of-view, the description of aspects of the visual field relative to the viewer. The other functions to analyze the relationship of one object to another in the visual field independent of the observer.[8] Each of these systems is strongly interconnected, existing in parallel in each cerebral hemisphere and processing the information from the contralateral eye. An operative cascade can be used to describe the cognitive processes involved in imagery—visual processing occurring without actual perceptual input (Fig. 7.1). This operative cascade has been adapted to filmmaking systems utilized in cinematography.

Beyond these systems utilized in conscious visual control, a major subcortical system functions at a nonconscious level to control eye movements and crossmodal spatial processes at speeds faster than those required for conscious mental processing. This independently functioning subcortical system, sometimes called the "visual buffer" can be manipulated, inducing us to focus our attention on part of an image or lead us to

1) Picture–develop your pattern and configuration map of the image,

2) Find–use attention to shift image properties and coordinate patterns,

3) Put–focus on the description and relationship of a part to the whole image, Image –establish object names, size, location, orientation and level of detail,

4) Resolution and re-generation–delineate the comparative detail of this image,

5) Look-for–integrate relevant memories,

6) Scan, zoom, pan and rotate–your presence, your operative attention in the image,

7) Answer-if–do properties associated with the image answer an already developed cognitive search parameter?

**Figure 7.1** The operative cascade of imagery.[13]

disengage from a representation. The most powerful triggers for this system are emotional stimuli that can change our focus and attention to a specific part of the visual field or to a visual representation stored in associative memory that was not part of the initial image.[14] A form of the subconscious visual buffer is also present in dreaming. Components of dream imagery can quickly "grab" our mental attention, reminiscent of the way it is subconsciously grabbed by emotionally competent stimuli during perception. Central (contextual) images of sufficient emotional import can trigger associated memories, co-opting the plot line of the dream. Emotion-associated dream images are those most likely to be remembered in waking.[15]

The visual neuroprocessing system is an operative system controlled by interconnected transmission line neural process connections and nuclear control sites. The operative cascade of visual imagery can be recreated in the process of filmmaking by the cinematographer. Such a mechanistic system can be recreated artificially with the described interconnections of this system closely resembling those of complex electronic systems.

Filmmakers have discovered other ways to manipulate this system of conscious visual processing, beyond the repetitive presentation of still images perceived as continuous. The viewer perceives cohesive objects as capable of tracing only one potential path through both space and time. Since real-world objects are rarely visualized in the static condition, we project viewed images along a potential trajectory before that sequence is ever shown. In a constructed film scene, the viewer follows characters and objects along an arc of motion even when obstructed from view, visually extrapolating progressions of actions to final results. We extend that process into our perspective of the plot, anticipating the conse-quences of actions and events.[16,17] Motion can include changes in both color and form. The brain registers the change in color first, before regis-tering the change in direction of motion, as based on the different proces-sing speed required for each of these cognitive systems to integrate perceptual input. The sensory visual cognitive process can also be manip-ulated in the way in which we perceive physical space. Renaissance artists learned to present spatial elements in a picture by mimicking the exact geometrical relationship of how light would meet the eye in a three-dimensional scene producing a consistent system so that a realistic appear-ance in depth and space could be achieved by the artist for the viewer. Perspective became the manner in which three-dimensional space was represented on a two-dimensional canvas. Visual presentation in photog-raphy, art, or film is most often viewed and judged based on the effects that changes in viewing angle, height, motion, and distance have on the viewer's perspective.[18]

## REPRESENTATIONAL IMAGES

The human CNS is, at its most basic level, a digital system con-structed of on—off neurons that either fire or don't fire. This operative aspect of neuron functioning can be described digitally as 01010.... Photographic images as originally developed were analogue in nature, the metaphoric imprint of light on chemically impregnated films. Television, as originally developed, was an intermediate form composed of on—off pixels that could be projected to fool our visual system into seeing a con-tiguous image. Today photography, television, and film have become digi-tal, constructed on large data collections based on the same 01010... coding. Such data are presented digitally as a picture. It is the viewer that converts this digitally presented data into analogue format.

Unsurprising, neurologic research compiled in recent decades suggests that our brains operate in a similar digital → analogue fashion. In the CNS, on—off patterns of neural firing are used to create internal analogue representations of experienced or conceived images. This internal display approximates on networks of nerve cells the visual form of an object anal-ogous to the visually perceived object. Such images exist in the brain as neural network images. Waking perceptual vision and imagery utilize these shared patterns of representational images to form an internal "I-language" of visual processing that we can use in responding to the visual complexity of the external world. Approximately half of the visual processing areas in the brain are topographically organized so as to represent externally perceived space and objects.[19,20,21] At these brain sites, the shared representational constructs that we use to process visual information exist virtually as visual constructs. These images comprise a system of internal coding utilized in our intrinsic memory system. When we look at an object and describe it as a "chair," that perception is based on our intrinsic memory for chair—the attributes that apply to many objects viewed from different perspectives that are all chairs.[22] Shared codes function in social interaction so that what you know as a chair is also what I see as a chair. Intrinsic representations, sometimes called "representational primitives," do not necessarily need to be learned, and are likely part of our genetic endowment. We use these representations to integrate the external images derived from perception with higher-order cognitive systems in the CNS. We use such representational primitives to categorize surfaces, and events (the temporal analogues for objects). Each of these categories of "primitive" has specific parameters, relationships, and transformations that govern its relation to other primitives. For instance, surface has parameters of "color," "depth," "texture," and "orientation," as well as relationship aspects of "junction," "edges," "concavities," "convexities," "gaps," and "holes."[23] Visual sensory input provides the triggering clues that activate the specific surface, object, and event codes that we then use to categorize, process, and theoretically group phenomena forming a visual I-grammar/syntax that can be used to structure the relationships between multiple and overlapping representations of objects, surfaces, and events. Multipart images utilize spatial relationships, the global shape or part of a shape of forms to create an overall image. The visual continuity of complex objects is maintained neurologically by relationships described as "binding." The different types of visual binding include: (1) property binding—different properties such as shape, color, and motion are bound to the objects that they characterize, (2) part binding—the parts of an object are segregated from the background and bound together, (3) range binding—particular values of a property such as color are defined within the dimension of that property, (4) hierarchical binding—the features of shape-defining boundaries are bound to the surface-defining properties of that object, (5) conditional binding—the interpretation of one property (e.g., motion) depends on another (e.g., depth, occlusion, or transparency), (6) temporal binding—successive states of the same object are integrated across temporal intervals as in real or apparent motion, and (7) location binding—in which objects are bound to their locations.[24] These properties are those utilized by editors and directors to create for the viewer a visually coherent film.

Mental images are not simple re-embodiments of stored sensory data. They exist for only a short time, developing and fading at a slower and more controlled rate, while the external objects of waking perception persist as long as they are present. The images incorporated into dream and imagery (nonperceptual imagery as utilized in eyes closed in waking) are limited by the information encoded into memory. We can exert control over the objects in these images while the external world is most often outside our volitional control. And, while depictive representations of the external environment include all aspects of shape, relationships to shape, color, texture, and spatial relationships in the visual field, propositional mental representations are abstract, often referring to classes of objects rather than a specific object.[13] This visual information is organized so that it can be utilized in the CNS for higher-level cognitive processing. The aspects of consciousness that can be attached to such images include an individual's associated memories, emotions, beliefs, attributions, and expectations.[25]

Dream imagery utilizes the same underlying systems of neural processing that are utilized in waking visual sensory perception.[12] But during dreaming, the representational imagery system has cognitive prominence. Dreams are most often a series of visual scenes, each comprised of representational images, tied together into narrative forms that utilize the internal formats (I-languages and grammar) of both thought and vision. While some of these representational images are mundane, object representations such as "chair," or "horse," others can be philosophically and spiritually profound: archetypical tidal waves, circles that could be the centers of the soul, or burning fires that can be interpreted as representations of an individual's god or devil. The dreamer is present in almost all dreams, most often as the point of view, the perspective from which the dream is observed. Most dreaming imagery is egocentric in nature, occurring to the left, to the right, in front of, or behind the dreamer. This egocentricity includes a general sense of one's body as a bounded object located within a space containing other objects. Dreams are often in motion, with the field of the image or a portion of the image altered under the direction of the dreamer. Image controls active during dreaming include the tendency to follow through to the completion of motions, the ability to scan and zoom in on an image, the ability to variably focus on the dreamscape, as well as the integration and manipulation of objects in relation to one another. Dream images are emotionally and cognitively penetrated. They include an individual's beliefs, attributions, or expectations regarding a particular mental image. These images can be combined and altered to produce creatively unexpected emergent forms. The thought space of dream imagery is very different from the visual perception of sensory space.[26] Dream images, although they appear to be images from the real world, are actually two-dimensional. Perceptions based on images from the external world have a vitality and vivacity that such nonperceptual imagery lacks. As Jean-Paul Sartre (1991) observed, if the object we select to imagine is the face of a close friend, one known in intricate detail, it will be, by comparison with an actual face, "thin," "dry," "two-dimensional," and "inert."[27] The narrative artist Eileen Scarry in her workshops likes to ask attendees to visualize a rose with their eyes closed. After several minutes she has them open their eyes and look at an actual rose. The difference is remarkable. Relative to the actual rose, the virtual rose of mental imagery is most often a pale and translucent reflection[28] (Fig. 7.2).

This topographically projected system is visually analogous to the linguistic concept of semiotic signs.[29] This concept of representational, metaphorical signs can be interpreted from the perspective of dream-based

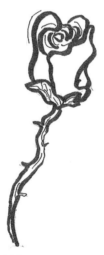

**Figure 7.2** A virtual rose of mental imagery.

archetypes and models developed by Carl Jung.[30] Contextual and shared Jungian archetypes are in many ways equivalent to the representational primitives that we use to define intrinsic visual and cognitive systems of perceptual interpretation. This system, cognitively active during both waking and sleeping consciousness utilizes same images that we use in intrinsic memory—our shared perceptual understandings of objects in the external world.[10] As Jung points out, any changes induced in these systems can alter a wide and pervasive range of consciousness and behavior, including personal psychodynamics and social projections. The filmmaker can manipulate representational images even to the point of portraying objects that were never intended to be representations (e.g., objects in stained walls and/or overlapping images that can be read as Rorschach blots). We process these powerfully contextual images within our own memory system, bringing our own history of experience, dreams, and associations into our role as a viewer so that what we see and experience can sometimes have little to do with the intentions and expectations of the filmmaker.

## DREAM MEMORIES

The images and thoughts in dream are derived from internal memories of waking experience. This in part accounts for the strong tendency for dream content to have continuity with our waking lives. These memories are incorporated into dreams and daydreams, plans, evaluations, and reasoning that takes place covertly. Most such internal cognitive experiences never result in observable actions or externally identifiable responses.[31] This makes such processes difficult to study. We do know, however, that different forms of memory are involved at different levels of the dream process:

1. Real memories of experienced events are incorporated and represented within the dream, contributing to dream content;
2. Memory processes functioning within the dream to organize, sequence, and monitor the dream narrative;
3. The dreamer upon awakening remembers the dream; and
4. The ways in which the dream is used in the dreamer's waking activities are affected by the intensity and persistence in the memory.[32]

Not long after the discovery of REM sleep, connections were discovered between sleep and memory processing.[33] The role of sleep in learning and in the consolidation of long-term memory is one of only a few of the proposed functions for sleep that is supported by experimental evidence.[34,35] Our long-term memories are generally divided into declarative memories under focused waking control (semantic memory (our factual knowledge of the world) and episodic memory (the contextual location of that memory in time and space)), and nondeclarative memories learned without conscious awareness (procedural memory (the learning of skills and habits, priming, classic conditioning), and at least two dream-associated memory forms (emotional and intrinsic memory)).[36] Different stages of sleep are involved in different kinds of memory.[37] The non-REM sleep stages are involved in the consolidation of explicit declarative learning.[38] The association of disordered REM sleep with PTSD supports a role for REM sleep dream function in nondeclarative emotionally charged memory processing.[39] It is less clear whether the cognitive process of dreaming has a role in learning or in the consolidation of memory. Viewed independently of sleep stage association, dream content can reflect recent learning, and may be helpful in creating new approaches to problem solving, but there is minimal evidence that dreaming reflects or contributes to memory consolidation.[40]

The cognitive architecture required for the transfer of imagery into conscious awareness requires interacting memory processes, the same systems that we use to process our sensory perceptions of external reality. A dream trace is often available for only seconds for potential incorporation into long-term memory stores. This short-term memory trace, often called working memory, utilizes the representational image/symbol system. Long-term memories are stored as synaptic networks or "kernals" of associated neural connections in specific areas of the brain (primarily the hippocampus).[41]

In connectionist AI models, memory can also be stored based on patterns of activation over a series of interconnected data storage nodes.[42] Such computer data storage systems can be organized in an attention-focused goal-based fashion to provide data access for system decision-making.[43] Such an interconnected, connectionist-based memory storage provides an ideal construct from which to develop the associated, meandering, and often creative associative image and thought memories that are incorporated into the content of dreams.[44] Attempts to incorporate quantum state variability mechanics into machine systemsare based at least in part on the attempt to approximate the patterns of biologic memory, including access to the genetic memory systems stored in cell nuclei DNA.[45]

## DREAM EMOTIONS

Emotions are the third of the primary cognitive processes that constitute dreams. A nonemotional dream is a none-sequitur on the same level as a state of living nonconsciousness. Even for individuals with disorders of emotion such as alexithymia, the decreased amount of emotion in dream reports is secondary to their dreams' continuity with their waking life of decreased emotion and their discomfort with reporting such experiences during dream recall.[46] Various lists of the emotions include pleasure, pain, elation, euphoria, ecstasy, sadness, desire, hope, aversion, despondency, depression, fear, contentment, anxiety, surprise, anger, and hostility. These mental experiences form the "bedrock of our minds" affecting and coloring all of our actions and thought.[47] Neurophysiologically, emotion has four major characteristics:

1. Experiences and perceptions that acquire emotional significance can become "emotionally competent stimuli;"
2. Once a stimulus acquires emotional significance, a pattern of autonomic and motor responses is triggered;
3. Circuits in the cerebral cortex are then triggered that process the associated feelings (the associated conscious sensations); and
4. Feedback from the peripheral, autonomic, and skeletomotor systems of emotional expression interact with conscious states of feeling in the cerebral cortex.[48]

Emotional expressions and feelings are controlled by distinct neuronal circuits, and mediated in the hippocampus, an area that also plays an important role in the processing of memory. Feelings are processed in the limbic system, a group of interconnected brain sites that includes the amyglada that has strong interconnections with cortical centers in the frontal, cingulate, and parahippocampal cortices of the cerebral cortex. This system is a repository for neural networks of specific emotional memories. Emotion-associated feelings can be viewed as our internal "perceptions" of these maps. In neurologically processing feelings, we utilize the same CNS systems that are used in processing external sensations or *qualia*—sensory qualities of the environment (the color red, the smell of coffee).[47] This CNS emotional processing system is integrated and connected with sensory and perceptual systems; CNS memory, processing, and integrating systems; and with the extensive networks of motor, sympathetic, endocrine, and parasympathetic expression that extend thoughout the body.

Emotion is sometimes the primary characteristic of the remembered dream. It is more likely to be negative than positive, so that cross-culturally, and for both men and women, dream content includes more aggression than friendliness, and more misfortune than good fortune.[49] The intensely experienced negative emotions of anxiety, fear, terror, anger, rage, embarrassment, and disgust can be profound and disturbing experiences, those typically associated with nightmares. Nightmares are the most commonly experienced of negative dreams. Intense negative emotions are also characteristically associated with other dreams and parasomnias including hypnagogic hallucinations at sleep onset, PTSD nightmares, and sleep paralysis that occur in sleep onset and REM sleep, and the night terrors and confusional arousals occurring in deep sleep.

The detection, generation, maintenance, and remembering of fear—the primary negative emotion—neuroanatomically takes place in four primary areas of the CNS operating in concert: the amygdala, the medial prefrontal cortex, the hippocampus, and the anterior cingulate cortex. Imaging studies indicate that these areas have increased activity during REM sleep, leading to proposals that nightmares occur secondary to the failure of a system of fear-memory extinction that functions during REM sleep dreaming.[50,51] Nightmares, the most common symptom of PTSD, occur after the experience of a trauma of such indigestible intensity as to break down our normally effective "protective shields," suggesting that emotional processing functioning during normal dreaming is overwhelmed by such trauma.[52] But emotional content, sometimes extreme in nature, is a component of dreaming from all sleep stages. All dreams, not just nightmares, are likely to have a functional role in the processing of the emotions associated with negative life experiences.

The subconscious visual buffer system is especially sensitive to emotional stimuli. As an example, emotion attached to an image can qualify that image as an emotionally competent stimulus able to affect the visual buffer, emotions, feelings, and even the dreams in which these images are combined and altered to produce unexpected emergent forms.[53] Such cognitive penetration can alter an image so that the image is processed in collateral cognitive processing systems.

Emotional expression is well within the capacity of AI systems, especially those with robotic capabilities. The automated version of the teddy bear ("tickle me Elmo") is a prime example, as is the smiley face utilized by the IBM Watson to improve the interface experience and accessibility as well as to reduce viewer frustration. Some AI specialists have contended that the ability to develop and maintain an emotional interface with a human is the marker for machine consciousness. Some contend that emotion and consciousness are not separable.[54] Emotional expressions are, however, easily copied and produced in a manner that humans, especially young humans, will respond to in very human ways, despite an absence of associated feelings in the system producing those emotional expressions. Researchers have cataloged and utilized facial recognition software to describe more than 2000 facial expressions as indicators for emotional states.[55] Purely reactive robots are being designed to set their entire behavior patterns in reaction to the external environment, so that the robot is under the control of the external environment. Emotions can be used by resource-limited AI systems as markers that permit new data and motive to get through protective filters, symbolic structures to be produced, preserved, or prevented.[56] For such a robot the sensory analysis of external emotions can be analyzed as motive generators. Detected emotional triggers utilized to develop internal representations (feelings?) can potentially lead to the self-generation of a mental life.[57]

Mood/emotion is within the capacity of artificial systems when defined as increases in persistent or motivated behaviors (good mood). Better (good) system mood levels are associated with higher execution speed and the self-selection of goals of increasing difficulty. Good mood in these studies is more likely to be present as a response to static and predictable environments in which there is a high chance to succeed. Lower mood states occur in response to a dynamic, high-difficulty environment with lower chances of success.[58] There are potential risks in using such emotional correlates for machine systems. The situation can be envisaged in which an armed computer-controlled drone, similar to systems in current use, chooses its target based on the presence of that target in a static environment in which there is high chance for a successful kill—a situation of high AI mood.

## CREATING THE ARTIFICIAL DREAM—NARRATIVE AND DIRECTION

Filmmaking is within the capacity of AI systems—the ability to create simulacrum dreamscapes that include the components that comprise a biologic dream. The limitations in this process are not technological. While complex, the technical paradigms of the dreaming brain: digital on−off neuron connections, memory storage, visual operative processing, interactive messaging systems, and emotional triggering/buffering systems operating at subliminal speeds, can or could be artificially constructed. The limitations of this process are rather based on the limits of our human understanding of the dream state. In its most basic form, a reported dream describes the way that we organize experience. This is not something that needs to be taught. Almost any human, even a small child, that has the capacity to communicate (language and social structure), will report their dreams as a narrative structure presented as a story. We structure our dream reports using the same methods and principles that we use for structuring waking thought. Dreams have other characteristics beyond the components of imagery, emotion, and memory. These components are formed into a narrative structure that forms an arc, often many arcs, in the process of developing a bidirectional and interactive story. This dream context of narrative structure is both easier and harder to artificially create.

Longer dream reports almost always have a clear narrative structure—a beginning, a middle, and an end. Narratives, subject to instant revision, are in a constant unstable motion that can both foreshorten and expand the dream experience. Most dreams have a plot—a continually evolving process of imagery and events. But that plot is loosely structured. Being interpersonal, dream reports can disregard the requirements of communicability and performance that are necessary for most stories. When confronted with someone else's report of their last night's dream, it is often difficult for the recipient of that report to maintain interest. The reported dream is most often a story with something missing.[10,59]

Today's films, cinematographic images created within the context of film narrative and sound, are coded representations of an external reality. The two processes (dreams and film) are clearly interactive. Images from the films that we watch are incorporated into our dreaming based on continuity with our lives, personal resonance, and the strength of the emotional stimuli.[60] In sharing a filmatic dream the filmmaker's interior world is projected onto the screen. That dream affects others, the viewers, the external society, and the culture.[61] The film viewer in watching film has learned to maintain the unstated awareness of watching a perceptual illusion that pretends to be real. The spatial parameters of visual shots are embedded within causal logic with transitions between shots disguised by the filmmaker and ignored by the viewer so that the images and sounds are experienced as a continuous present moving forward in time. This is a technically defined process. Narrative flow can be altered and expanded with editing, since editing, like cinematography, is based on, adapted to, and reflective of an operative cascade (Fig. 7.1). Master shots brought together in parallel and then into focus can be used to bring together disparate tracks of the story line. Detail shots internalize psychological themes and structures for the viewer. Interjected flashbacks take the narrative back in time from the current point. While the director of a film may attempt to subvert our expectations of narrative, genre, pace, time, and character, once the story fits within a defined narrative structure, it is difficult to subvert an audience's expected illusion. The interplay between filmmaker and audience becomes a dance of expectations that are only sometimes fulfilled. It was Freud's apparatus theory that first suggested that remembered dreams and the unconscious mind could operate within the dynamic of filmmaking. Post-Freudians suggested that filmmakers affect us emotionally and alter our perceptual view of the exterior universe by accessing the same mental systems that we utilize in our dreams. Filmmakers have developed complex methods of storytelling based on this perspective. Jacque Lacan called this process "suture," a medically based metaphor implying that through techniques such as editing, a film could be "sewn" shut so as to include the viewer.[62] The sutured viewer shifts from one character or scene to another following the eye-lines (gaze) of the characters, accepting what is seen on film from multiple perspectives and directions as natural and personally impactful. In the classic example of shot/reverse shot editing, two characters are viewed alternatively over the other's shoulder. We do not ask "Who is watching?" because each shot answers the question of the previous shot. We as viewers adopt the point-of-view of dream vicariously becoming each character we are watching. The projected dream of cinema is an intentionally accepted delusion experienced when awake, with the viewer enmeshed into a film "reality" in an imaginary present tense.[63]

Film images are propositional forms, outlines rather than fully formed images that are very similar to representational primitives. In our brains, these images change even more quickly than the presented stills of a moving picture, appearing and disappearing at the speed of thought on a millisecond to millisecond basis, creating a synthetic temporal dimension tied into an awareness of our own life experience. During both film and dreaming the emotionally competent visual buffer functions as a varyingly conscious cognitive interface. The films that we watch lead us down a Purkinji tree of associated image, thought, and emotional memories, just as in dreaming. In our viewing or reading the constructed dream, we interject our own memories, emotions, and imagery into the experience. And once enmeshed, once sutured into the inner world of that scene and that character, our cognitive experience extends beyond the experience of the artificial dreamscape. The filmmaker can entice the viewer into a vicarious experience that resembles less a dream and more the vivacity of actual experience.[64] But, we as viewers experience something far different than what was designed or plotted by the writer. The viewer is an onlooker to his own dream, enveloped by the presented dream just as a child is enveloped by his world. The subject does not see where a dream is leading yet he/she follows into a worldview that is often filled with unexplainable magic.[65]

## AI-CREATED DREAMS

Storytelling can be magic. Filmmaking illuminates that magic with the technical capacity to incorporate images, acted emotions, and sounds into a narrative structure. As noted repeatedly in this book, that which can be described can be technically created. For our species the need to record dreams has been a consistent pattern recorded in our oldest artifacts and our earliest decipherable attempts at writing. With the development of each new technology used to record or create, the first documented attempts in that medium have often been attempts to recreate dreams. There is little question that artificially created films, simulacrums of dreaming, are within the technical capacity of AI systems. In order to cogently interact with humans at the interface, these systems are very likely to comprise the next generation of filmmakers.

## Notes

1. Freud, S. (1914). Remembering, repeating and working-through. In J. Strachey (Ed.), *The standard edition of the complete psychological works* (Vol. V, p. 511). London: Hogarth Press.
2. British Film Institute and National Film Archive (Great Britain). *Early cinema: Primitives and pioneers (1895–1910)*. London: BFI Video Publishing.

3. Rodowick, D. N. (1997). *Giles Deleuze's time machine.* Durham, NC: Duke University Press.
4. Klatsky, R., & Lederman, S. (1993). Spatial and non-spatial avenues to object recognition by the human haptic system. In N. Eilan, R. McCarthy, & B. Brewer (Eds.), *Philosophy and psychology* (pp. 191–205). Oxford: Oxford Press.
5. Cartwright, R., Bernick, N., Borowitz, G., & Kling, A. (1969). Effects of an erotic movie on the dreams of young men. *Archives of General Psychiatry, 20,* 263–271.
6. Ullman, M., & Limmer, C. (Eds.). (1988). *The variety of dream experience.* New York: Continuum; Buckley, K. (1996). *Among all those dreamers: Essays on dreaming in modern society.* Albany, NY: State University of New York Press.
7. Kosslyn, S., Thompson, W., & Ganis, G. (2006). *The case for mental imagery* (pp. 13–14). Oxford and New York: Oxford University Press.
8. Gregory, R. (1997). *Eye and brain: The psychology of seeing* (pp. 76–77). Princeton, NJ: Princeton University Press.
9. Zeki, S., & Bartels, A. (1999). Toward a theory of visual consciousness. *Consciousness and Cognition, 8,* 225–259.
10. Pagel, J. F. (2014). *Dream science: Exploring the forms of consciousness.* Oxford: Academic Press.
11. Finke, R., & Shepard, R. (1986). Visual functions of mental imagery. In K. Boff, L. Kaufman, & J. Thomas (Eds.), *Handbook of perception and human performance* (p. 37). New York: Wiley-Interscience.
12. Thompson, W., & Kosslyn, S. (2000). Neural systems activated during visual mental imagery: A review and meta-analysis. In A. Toga & J. Mazziotta (Eds.), *Brain mapping: The systems* (pp. 535–560). San Diego, CA: Academic Press.
13. Kosslyn, S. (1994). *Image and brain: The resolution of the imagery debate. Bradford book.* Cambridge, MA: The MIT Press.
14. Vuilleumier, P., & Swartz, S. (2001). Beware and be aware: Capture of spatial attention by fear-related stimuli in neglect. *NeuroReport, 12,* 1119–1122.
15. Kuiken, D., & Sikora, S. (1993). The impact of dreams on waking thoughts and feelings. In A. Moffitt, M. Kramer, & R. Hoffman (Eds.), *The functions of dreaming* (pp. 419–476). Albany, NY: State University of New York Press.
16. Eilen, N., McCarthy, R., & Brewer, B. (Eds.). (1993). *Spatial representation: Problems in philosophy and psychology.* Oxford: Oxford University Press.
17. Zeki, S. (1999). *Inner vision: An exploration of art and the brain* (pp. 66–67). Oxford: Oxford University Press.
18. Mausfield, R. (2003). Conjoint representations. In H. Hetch, R. Schwartz, & M. Atherton (Eds.), *Looking into pictures: An interdisciplinary approach to pictorial space* (pp. 17–60). Cambridge, MA: The MIT Press.
19. Fox, P., Mintum, M., Raichle, M., Miezin, F., Allman, J., & Van Essen, D. (1986). Mapping human visual cortex with positron emission tomography. *Nature, 323,* 806–809.
20. Felleman, D., & Van Essen, D. (1991). Distributed hierarchical processing in primate cerebral cortex. *Cerebral Cortex, 1,* 1–47.
21. Sereno, M., Pitzalis, S., & Martinez, A. (2001). Mapping of contralateral space in retinotopic coordinates by a parietal cortical area in humans. *Science, 294,* 1350–1354.
22. Roediger, H., Weldon, M., & Challis, B. (1989). Explaining dissociations between implicit and explicit measures of retention: A processing account. In F. Dempster & C. Brainerd (Eds.), *Interference and cognition* (pp. 29–59). New York: Academic Press Inc.
23. Mausfeld, R. (2003). Conjoint representations and the mental capacity for multiple simultaneous perspectives. In H. Hecht, R. Schwartz, & M. Atherton (Eds.), *Looking into pictures: An interdisciplinary approach to pictorial space* (pp. 32–33). Cambridge, MA: The MIT Press.

24. Treisman, A. (2000). The binding problem. In L. Squire & S. Kosslyn (Eds.), *Findings and current opinion in cognitive neuroscience* (pp. 31–38). Cambridge, MA: The MIT Press.

25. Finke, R. (1990). *Creative imagery: Discoveries and inventions in visualization.* Hillsdale, NJ: Erlbaum.

26. States, B. (1997). *Seeing in the dark: Reflections on dreams and dreaming* (p. 97). New Haven, NJ: Yale University Press.

27. Sartre, J. (2004). *The imaginary: A phenomenological psychology of the imagination* (J. Webber, Trans.). London and New York: Routledge (Original work published 1940).

28. Scary, E. (1995). On vivacity: The difference between daydreaming and imagining-under-authorial-instruction. *Representations, 52,* 1–26.

29. "A sign is a picture if the perception of the essential properties that the sign has in relevant respects is identical to the perception one would have of the corresponding properties of some other object under a certain perspective and if this perception is constitutive for the interpretation of the sign" Sachs-Hombach, K. (2003). Resemblance reconceived. In H. Hetch, R. Schwartz, & M. Atherton (Eds.), *Looking into pictures: An interdisciplinary approach to pictorial space* (pp. 167–178). Cambridge, MA: The MIT Press.

30. Jung, C. (1974). On the nature of dreams. In *Dreams* (R. Hull, Trans., p. 68). Princeton, NJ: Princeton University Press (Original work published 1948).

31. Cohen, G. (1996). *Memory in the real world* (p. 22). Hove: Psychology Press.

32. Pagel, J. F., & Vann, B. (1997). Cognitive organization of dream mentation: Evidence for correlation with memory processing systems. *ASDA Abstracts.*

33. Pagel, J. F., Pegram, V., Vaughn, S., Donaldson, P., & Bridgers, W. (1973). REM sleep and intelligence in mice. *Behavioral Biology, 9,* 383–388.

34. Walker, M. (2005). A refined model of sleep and the time course of memory formation. *Behavioral and Brain Sciences, 28,* 51–104.

35. Squire, L. (2004). Memory systems in the brain: A brief history and current perspective. *Neurobiology of Learning and Memory, 82,* 171–177.

36. Siegel, J. (2005). The incredible shrinking sleep-learning connection. *Behavioral and Brain Sciences, 28,* 82–83; Vertes, R. (2005). Sleep is for rest, waking consciousness is for learning and memory—of any kind. *Behavioral and Brain Sciences, 28,* 86–87.

37. Stickgold, R., Hobson, J., Fosse, R., & Fosse, M. (2001). Sleep, learning and dreams: Off-line memory processing. *Science, 294,* 1052–1057.

38. Stickgold, R., James, L., & Hobson, J. (2000). Visual discrimination learning requires sleep after training. *Nature Neuroscience, 3,* 1237–1238.

39. Levin, R., Fireman, G., & Nielsen, T. (2010). Disturbed dreaming, and emotional dysregulation. In J. F. Pagel (Ed.), *Dreaming and nightmares. Sleep medicine clinics* (Vol. 5, pp. 229–240). Philadelphia, PA: Saunders.

40. Smith, C. (2010). Sleep states, memory processing, and dreams. In J. F. Pagel (Ed.), *Dreaming and nightmares. Sleep medicine clinics* (Vol. 5, pp. 217–228). Philadelphia, PA: Saunders.

41. Kandel, E. (2000). Cellular mechanisms of learning and the biological basis of individuality. In E. Kandel, J. Schwartz, & T. Jessell (Eds.), *Principles of neural science* (4th ed., pp. 1247–1312). New York: McGraw-Hill.

42. Sun, R. (2014). Connectionism and neural networks. In K. Frankish & W. Ramsey (Eds.), *The Cambridge handbook of artificial intelligence* (pp. 108–127). Cambridge: Cambridge University Press.

43. Taylor, J. (2007). Through machine attention to machine consciousness. In A. Chella & R. Manzotti (Eds.), *Artificial consciousness* (pp. 24–47). Charlottesville, VA: Imprint Academic.

44. Stickgold, R. (2003). Memory, cognition and dreams. In P. Maguet, C. Smith, & R. Stickgold (Eds.), *Sleep and brain plasticity* (pp. 17–39). Oxford: Oxford Press.

45. Kelly, K. (2010). *What technology wants* (pp. 307–309). New York: Viking.
46. Lumley, M., & Bazydlo, R. (2000). The relationship of alexithymia characteristics to dreaming. *Journal of Psychosomatic Research, 48*, 561–567.
47. Damasio, A. (2003). *Looking for Spinoza: Joy, sorrow and the feeling brain* (p. 3). Orlando, FL: Harcourt, Inc.
48. Iverson, S., Kupfermann, I., & Kandel, E. (2000). Emotional states and feelings. In E. Kandel, J. Swartz, & T. Jessell (Eds.), *Principles of neural science* (4th ed., p. 982). New York: McGraw-Hill.
49. Domhoff, G. W. (2003). *The scientific study of dreams: Neural networks, cognitive development, and content analysis* (p. 26). Washington, DC: American Psychological Association.
50. Levin, R., & Nielsen, T. (2007). Disturbed dreaming, posttraumatic stress disorder, and affect distress: A review and neurocognitive model. *Psychological Bulletin, 133*, 482–528.
51. Nofzinger, E. (2004). What can neuroimaging findings tell us about sleep disorders. *Sleep Medicine, 5*(Suppl 1), S16–S22.
52. Freud, S. (1951). *Beyond the pleasure principle: Vol 18. The standard edition* (J. Strachey, Trans. & Ed.). London: Hogarth (Original work published 1916).
53. Pagel, J. F., Kwiatkowski, C., & Broyles, K. (1999). Dream use in film making. *Dreaming, 9*(4), 247–296.
54. Damasio, A. (1999). *The feeling of what happens: Body and emotion in the making of consciousness* (p. 16). San Diego, CA: Harcourt Inc.
55. Ekman, P. (2007). *Emotions revealed* (2nd ed.). New York: Owl Books.
56. Sloman, A. (2005). Motive, mechanisms and emotions. In M. Boden (Ed.), *The philosophy of artificial intelligence* (pp. 232–233). Oxford: Oxford University Press.
57. Parasi, D. (2007). Mental robotics. In A. Chella & R. Manzotti (Eds.), *Artificial consciousness* (pp. 191–211). Charlottesville, VA: Imprint-Academic.
58. Caci, B., Cardaci, M., Chella, A., D'Amacio, A., Infantino, I., & Macaluso, I. (April 12–15, 2005). Personality and learning in robots. The role of individual motivations/expectations/emotions in robot adaptive behaviors. In *Proceedings of the symposium "Agents that want and like: Motivational and emotional roots of cognition and action"*. Hatfield: University of Hertfordshire.
59. Hunt, H. (1989). *The multiplicity of dreams*. New Haven, CT: Yale University Press.
60. Cristie, I. (1994). *The last machine: Early cinema and the birth of the modern world*. London: British Film Institute.
61. Allen, R. (1995). *Projecting illusion-film spectatorship and the impression of reality* (p. 115). Cambridge: Cambridge University Press.
62. Lacan, J. (1979). The imaginary signifier. In *Four fundamental concepts of psychoanalysis* (A. Sheridan, Trans., p. 75). Harmondsworth: Penguin Books Ltd.
63. Friedberg, A. (1990). A denial of difference: Theories of cinematic identification. In E. Kaplan (Ed.), *Psychoanalysis and cinema* (p. 36). New York: Routledge.
64. Scarry, E. (1999). *Dreaming by the book*. Princeton, NJ: Princeton University Press.
65. Kaplan, A. (Ed.). (1990). *Psychoanalysis and cinema* (p. 7). New York: Routledge.

The relationship of filmmaking to dreaming is addressed in far more detail in the earlier books by this author (*The Limits of Dream* and *Dream Science*). Viewed in this manner, these books can be viewed as a series, addressing the history of dreams and dream study, the current status of the field outside REM sleep, and prospects for the future.

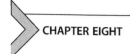

CHAPTER EIGHT

# The Cyborg at the Dream Interface

*Love of semiconductors is not enough. . .*

*Thomas Nagel (1994).[1]*

Humans evolved sensory and behavior interface capacities in order to interact with their external environment. Computer systems were originally developed in order to expand this interaction. Advances in both hardware and software have developed this interface into a direct extension of our senses and CNS capacity. Our modern existence has become increasingly dependent on such extensions. The human immersed in the interactive interface utilizes different perceptual capabilities, assesses alternative and extended mnemonic processing, and has different and expanded capacities for emotional, decision-making, and behavioral expression. Remarkable achievements can be attributed to this computer–human interface. With our capabilities expanded by computer assistance, we have been able to explore outer space, as well as the inner space of the basic scientific nature of existence.

Humans utilize genetically developed perceptual systems to produce a representational construct in interfacing with the external environment. This sensory construct is but one of many alternative possibilities. In our immediate biosphere, there are dogs with an extended aural and olfactory range, birds with differences in color vision, acuity, and frequency awareness, and fish with electromagnetic sensitivity and a visual system designed to function in a very different medium from air. Multiple organisms have evolved differently in order to suit their environment, utilizing chemical, electrical, and substrate sensors to produce a perspective of three-dimensional external space undeniably different from our own. Other dimensions, approachable in representation from the machine perspective, can be used to describe external space in an alternative spatial presentation that is difficult for those of us restricted to three-dimensions to cogently comprehend.

The interface between human and computer is also limited by our individual cognitive capacities, and our human interface requirements for

*Machine Dreaming and Consciousness.*
DOI: http://dx.doi.org/10.1016/B978-0-12-803720-1.00008-6

auditory, visual, numeric, and/or linguistic representations. The typical user cannot mentally retain or numerically integrate complex or large number groups, a capability that when required by a computer interface (as in the use of typical cryptogenic passwords) can produce a noninteractive state in which the interface is not operable.[2] Both our attentional and memory systems are time-based so that over time, humans forget much of learned information and behavior. Distractions and interruptions can negatively affect maintenance of the human—computer interaction. A similar pattern exists when one tries to remember or describe the previous night's dream.

Other functioning CNS systems involved in cognitive processing are less developed and involved in the environmental interface. Some of these systems are perceptual (e.g., nonconscious visual movement buffers). Other systems such as those involved in cognitive and mnemonic processing are functional during waking, but typically operating in a nonconscious manner (e.g., recall for the second to last letter of your middle name). Some of these systems cannot clearly be accessed in waking consciousness. They become apparent when addressed with well-designed behavioral testing (visual buffers), or when an effort of waking attention and focus is applied (middle name letters). Other systems, such as the CNS synchronous physiologic electrical field system, function throughout the CNS, yet operate outside conscious assessment. This nonconscious system forms a CNS electrophysiologic framework that may be the global platform on which consciousness operates.[3] It functions primarily during sleep—especially during the conscious states of sleep that include dreaming—and in unfocused waking. These nonconscious systems are described and assessed using computer-based monitoring systems, and as such, these systems are technically available for bidirectional assess. Today, we are extending our interface capacity into these nonperceptual systems.[4] Such changes in the interface will alter patterns of access. Computer systems will change, and how we use systems for sensory augmentation will change. In turn, so will we.

## KEYBOARD-BASED MACHINE INTERFACE SYSTEMS

Today, the computer keyboard is the primary input method used for interface interactions. Keyboard access is in the midst of rapid change. Different keys can be used to produce symbols having different meanings for different users (languages, grammars, and representations), and different meanings for the system being used (e.g., double clicking; a graphical interface system left on after discontinuation of drawing results in a disruption and change in writing format). Such alternative modal selection does expand the capacity of the keyboard, but it can also lead to modal confusion. Aircraft crashes have been attributed to such a modal confusion between the operator and the computer control system.[5] Graphical input devices—cursors, tap keys, and mice—have markedly expanded keyboard capacity for interaction. Hyperlink systems have expanded file, data, and Internet search program access. Short cuts, icons, functioning screensavers, and sleep modes can expand interface functioning. Each added function that contributes to system complexity increases the potential for interactional confusion. Human technical capacity at the keyboard interface has also expanded as conscious processes have become nonconscious (typing or thumb input), and simultaneous so that we are able to alternate our focused attention between tasks (texting and talking).[6]

## REACHING BEYOND THE KEYBOARD
### The auditory interface

Our auditory sensing system is designed to convert external frequency-based modulations conducted through the atmosphere into neuro-electrical signals that we interpret as sound. Frequencies ranging from 1 to 30 Hz can be "heard" by our auditory sensorium. Discrete beat patterns in lower-frequency ranges can be achieved on percussion instruments. The normal frequency that can be accomplished with rapid finger tapping is 10 beats/min (alpha).[7] Beats and frequencies in the physiologic range comprise much of what we refer to as "music," sounds that after electronic modulation, fill the soundscape of our modern world.

In the last few years auditory interface systems have become the norm. They are commonly used even in highly complex environments. Such systems use hierarchical pattern recognition systems to identify interpretable statements in human speech.[8] Auditory interface systems side-step potential keyboard errors but expand the potential for interactional malapropisms by adding linguistic confusion, altered noun–verb presentation, individual variability, and a required monotony of presentation.

For many years, direct attempts have been made to develop auditory sleep-associated teaching or hypnopedia. These attempts have met with minimal success.[9] There is good evidence, however, that some stimuli externally applied during sleep can affect both sleep-associated electrophysiology and dreaming. During lighter sleep (stage 1, 2, and REM sleep), the externally vocalized expression of the individual's name can induce either a microarousal or a K-complex in monitored sleep.[10] Aversive stimuli (the tightening of a blood pressure cuff, sounds, flashing lights) are sometimes incorporated into reported dream content.[11] It has been difficult to demonstrate the capacity for hypnopedia to induce more complex alterations in cognitive processing.

## The visual interface

Eyeglass-based screens (e.g., Google Glass) operate like cell phone screens using tracking pads that respond to three main finger gestures. Tap once to select. Slide your finger along the temples to scroll, or swipe down to dismiss a screen.[12] Eye tracking still holds great promise as a human—computer interface. In the early days, eye tracking was done with mechanical/optical instruments that tracked mirrored contact lens reflections, or instruments that measured eye muscle tension. Newer approaches illuminate the eye with infrared light and monitor reflected motion with a camera. But this approach has not been easy to apply. Eye focus physiologically wanders, rarely maintained in one site of focus for more than milliseconds, so that eye movement must be statistically modeled based on an aggregate assessment of eye motions that the eye uses to attend. Vertices of change in direction of eye movements can be used to better focus the locations of eye tracking that can be used to model the visual attention induced by social cues.[13] Each screen presented changes context for the user. Eye movement sensors can also be used to enable otherwise disabled individuals to have access to their computers. Visual interface systems can now capture images and translate those images internally in the CNS into retinal simulations. Some of these systems have provided sufficient visual information in otherwise blind patients to allow pattern and letter recognition.[14]

## Hardwiring: the direct human—machine interface

The plugged-in terminal man is a mainstay of futuristic scientific fiction. Currently interface systems can access, utilize, and adjust the constituents of our body's fluid reservoirs, providing real-time intravenous and interthecal chemical adjustments able to affect both physical and mental functioning. Prominent examples include glucose monitoring and adjustment of insulin dosages in type I diabetics, and medications for the treatment of intractable pain. Neurochemically psychoactive drugs such as opiates can be injected into serum or interthecally into spinal fluids in order to alter waking and sleeping behaviors.

Conceptually, direct plugged-in nerve interactions are based on the concept of transmission line neuroanatomy in which the human CNS is viewed as a hard-wired system of interconnected neural processes. While this is a primary level of CNS organization, it is simplistic, not addressing the complex neurochemical, neuroendocrine, and electrophysiological systems known to alter and effect CNS functioning. Direct neural interface is most easily applicable in the skeletal musculature where direct neural discharge-based behavioral analogues can be controlled with mechanical, computer-modulated devices. These systems are now a mainstay of replacement prosthesis technology. Directly applied computer-controlled induced electrical discharge systems have also been effectively used in treating Parkinson disease and intractable seizures.

Monitoring and implementation of the brain–computer interface (BCI) can be invasive or noninvasive, providing a new channel of output for the brain. Such a system requires the user to develop voluntary adaptive control in order to interact with the device. This interaction is enabled through a variety of intermediary functional components, control signals, and feedback loops.[15] Such systems can sometimes be remarkably simple. A robotic arm can be controlled in real time with the microwire-controlled electrical discharge at a single motor neuron. The direction of hand movement, gripping force, hand velocity, acceleration, and three-dimensional position can be derived using mathematic models in order for complex hand movements to be produced in response to arbitrary sensory cues.[16]

Sensory events can induce powerful electrical signals that overwhelm the background electrical activity of the EEG. These event-related potentials (ERPs) are time-locked, occurring at a fixed time after an external or internal event such as a sensory or aural stimulus, a mental event, or the omission of a constantly occurring stimulus. Types of ERPs are commonly used in BCI including the visual-evoked potential (VEP), an EEG component that occurs in response to a visual stimulus, and the P300, an endogenous ERP component that occurs after unexpected stimuli or the unexpected absence of an expected event.[17] The P300 is a repeatable, large positive wave that occurs approximately 300 ms after an event. Most training methods requiring the user to perform specific cognitive tasks focus on developing the user's ability to generate EEG components through voluntary, conscious mental activity. This P300 response is especially useful in cases where a user cannot be easily trained.[18]

Motor imagery tasks generate signals in the sensorimotor cortex of the brain that can be detected by EEG and used to modulate control of various tasks.[19] In contrast, operant conditioning focuses on teaching a behavior to the user based on feedback provided by the system. Both methods of training are affected by numerous external factors including concentration, distractions, frustration, emotional state, fatigue, motivation, intention, first/third-person perspective, visualization of the action versus retrieving a memory of the action performed earlier, and imagination of the task as opposed to a verbal narration. Fine details are difficult for either type of user to control.[20]

Attention is an important component of global brain states. The gamma EEG rhythm has been proposed as a binding marker for attentional consciousness.[21] As for most EEG rhythms, biofeedback can be used to train individuals to develop gamma activity.[22] Attempts to design BCI systems using gamma as a CNS marker of attention have been constrained by the effects of interference, sampling, and artifacts on scalp electrodes. Gamma biofeedback systems require that EEG electrodes be implanted inside the skull. Interface use of gamma has also been limited by the lack of any clear causal link connecting gamma oscillations with the processes of attentional information processing.[23]

## THE NEUROELECTRIC INTERFACE

Keyboard, auditory, and visual interface systems adapted to human sense and behavioral patterns, and controlled drug infusion systems are currently in widespread use. Direct-wired systems have demonstrated their usefulness in prosthesis control, as well as in visual and auditory replacements. Beyond these approaches, there are other systems that have the potential to extend the interface well beyond current capabilities. Frequency-based electrical fields are one example. This system operates on a millisecond-to-millisecond basis in the CNS, utilizing extracellular propagated electrical fields that affect neuron firing, ion-equilibrium at the cell membranes, intracellular kinetics, and potentially the DNA expression of genetic memory stores. The CNS systems that utilize these electrophysiologic fields in their functioning are primarily those involving associative memory, intrinsic imagery, and emotions—phenomenological components of dreaming.[24] Neurochemicals known to alter this system produce consistent patterns of behavioral change.[25] The external manipulation and/or application of external electrical fields can alter this system and affect the cognitive behaviors and memory processes that utilize this system. This system can be trained using biofeedback. The frequency patterns of these EEG fields are altered in individuals who regularly meditate.[26]

## Electroshock therapy (ECT and TMS)

Electroconvulsive therapy (ECT) has been used for many years to treat psychiatric disorders. The externally applied electrical fields are in excess of the physiologic range, usually 800 mA, up to several hundred watts, with current flows timed between 1 and 6 s. Today, ECT is usually applied as a pulsed direct current, since frequency modulated currents are more likely to result in memory disturbance.[27] Transcranial magnetic stimulation (TMS) is a more recently developed approach in which an externally applied magnetic field is used. The TMS field can pass unimpeded through skin and skull to induce a directed current in the brain, activating nearby nerve cells in much the same way as electrical currents when applied directly to the cortical surface.[28] Single or paired pulse TMS currents induce neurons under the site of stimulation to depolarize and discharge an action potential. When used in the occipital cortex, "phosphenes" (flashes of light) are sometimes reported. When used in most other areas of the cortex, the participant does not consciously experience any effect, yet behavior may be altered (e.g., slower reaction time on a cognitive task), and changes in brain activity may be detected.[29] When used to treat severe depression and psychosis, both ECT and TMS rival the efficacy that can be achieved with medication. Both approaches can also produce confusion and disturbances in memory.[27,29]

## Biofeedback

Since the early 1970s, biofeedback has been used to train individuals to develop physiologic brain rhythms. Individuals trained in developing the theta and alpha rhythms report relaxation and drowsiness.[30] EEG biofeedback training has proven beneficial for some patients in the treatment of epileptic seizures, learning disability, PTSD, chronic fatigue, tobacco dependence, and AD/HD.[31] In sports, performance, military, and artistic training, frequency-based biofeedback systems are sometimes used in the attempt to assist individuals to develop task focus. While many studies have shown individually positive results using this approach, a lack of technique consistency, patent controls of data, and underdeveloped methodology have made it difficult to determine the overall potential for this approach. Recently, EEG feedback has been incorporated into virtual reality and gaming systems.[32]

## Meditation

Individuals involved in long-term meditative practice often demonstrate changes in their EEG frequencies.[26] The changes in EEG activity recorded depend on the type of meditation technique used. The patterns of alpha and beta/gamma (33–44 Hz) band activity differ in focused mediators from what is found in individuals practicing unfocused meditation styles.[33] Tibetan techniques of meditation include training in the capacity to extend meditative focus into sleep—what some authors have proposed as a highly controlled form of lucid dreaming.[34] Lucid dreaming with signalling is a state incorporating wake-like alpha and beta/gamma activity that may be best conceptualized as a meditation-like state occurring during sleep rather than wake.[35]

## Environmental electrical fields

Without preparation and with little, if any, testing as to the potential physiologic and psychological effects, the human species has subjected itself to an external environment that is filled with the broadcast of strong frequency-modulated electrical fields. These fields are in the same frequency range as the physiological electrical fields that our brains use for multiple functions. Today it is the rare human who does not interface with 60 Hz alternating electric current on an almost full-time basis. Like all frequency-based electrical fields, it is broadcast into the surrounding space beyond the various components, wires, and systems that use it as a power source. In the hospital setting where EEG monitoring is utilized to document the lack of brain electrical activity (brain death), background 60 Hz electrical activity is invariably present as an "artifact" on EEG recordings. The effects induced by this external electrical field on the EEG can make the differential between "death" and "life" difficult to determine. In most cases, 60 Hz contamination can only be eliminated by the use of blocking filters that also technically eliminate some of the EEG frequencies in the physiologic range (beta and gamma)—the same frequencies that some propose as markers for consciousness. Surprisingly, humans seem to tolerate exposure to these electrical fields. Epidemiologically, there is little direct evidence that physiologic harm results from our ubiquitous exposure to 60 Hz. While there remain questions as to whether common diagnoses in our modern world (cancer, Alzheimer disease, anxiety, and depression) might be in some way tied to background electrical field exposure, there is minimal empiric evidence supporting this possibility.[36]

We subject ourselves less often to other externally propagated electrical frequencies known to affect CNS physiologic electrical systems. During the "Cold War," within the Soviet block nations, massive aversive weapon broadcast systems were built to broadcast alpha and other physiologic frequencies into North America and Western Europe. The largest of these systems, called "Duga," was constructed within the Chernobyl Complex in what is now the Ukraine. This "over-the-horizon" radar system was designed to have both offensive and defensive capacities. This immensely powerful broadcast system induced SOS call interference throughout Europe in the 10 Hz range. Short-wave sets had to be redesigned with blocking filters to eliminate this irritating interference, referred to in the popular press as the "Russian Wood-Pecker."[37] But despite this continuous application of external alpha frequency, the most dominant of our physiologic rhythms, there is little evidence for any adverse health or other physiologic effects induced by the exposure of millions of people to this broadcast field. Despite the lack of such evidence, there are some who believe that current European psychological and political disarray is in some way secondary to the recent reactivation of this system's broadcast into Europe from sites in western Russia.[38]

## Summary: the neuroelectric interface

The brain's electrophysiological system is affected and altered by externally applied chemicals and electrical fields, biofeedback, and entrained approaches to meditative practice. When external fields are applied in the supraphysiologic range electrically as ECT or magnetically as TMS, alterations in cognitive processing, memory and sensory systems are induced that can affect the course of a variety of psychiatric illnesses. While humans are routinely exposed to electrical and magnetic fields in the physiological ranges, the functional effects induced by these fields are limited, especially when compared to the effects that can be induced by interaction with visual and auditory sensory interface systems such as television, video gaming, and film.[39] It is unclear as to how the CNS electrophysiological system is able to protect itself from the exposure to these external environmental fields.

The electrophysiological interface differs in basic ways from the current systems utilizing waking perceptual processing:

1. These are nonsensory-based interactions;
2. Since biologically this system operates primarily in a nonconscious manner, any interface-induced alteration in this system is likely to have nonconscious expression;
3. The biologic and AI systems that utilize these electrical fields in their function include those involved in supplying energy, establishing ionic equilibrium, storing information, and communicating between widely separated or otherwise unconnected networks. These systems are most likely to be available to interface interaction;
4. This system is minimally or alternatively utilized in waking focused thought, and it will be difficult to demonstrate waking cognitive effects induced by interactive alterations in this system;
5. The cognitive changes induced by such an interface interaction are most likely to be apparent in those cognitive systems that utilize frequency-based electrical fields: waking mind-wandering, emotional and creative processing, and sleep-associated conscious processing (dreaming).

The frequency-based electrophysiologic system is one example of how the computer—human interface can be expanded beyond the typically utilized perceptual interactions. Cognitively, we typically utilize these electrophysiologic systems in non- or alternatively conscious functioning. The interface potential for this system is less likely to be on conscious waking thought, and more likely be on conscious states that utilize this system in cognitive functioning, such as those involved in dreaming and dream-like states. Dreams incorporate associative memory, intrinsic imagery, and emotions in executive processes including emotional processing and creative problem solving. These are the CNS systems that should be amenable to interaction with an electrophysiology-based interface.

The prospects for such alternatively conscious, broadcast interface systems are potentially profound. Independently of human input, AI systems utilize similar frequency-based electrical potentials to convey data, communicate, supply power, and to store neural net configurations. Today, we use electromagnetic operative frequency broadcast modes in cell-phone, and computer-to-computer communication. The activity of these systems produces electromagnetic ration akin to the brainwaves of the CNS. Human communication systems can be monitored and analyzed by artificial intelligence (AI) systems using capacities extending beyond the human biologic range. From both human and AI perspectives, this system has the potential to function more fully in human—machine interaction.

## THE DREAM INTERFACE

For the human, dreams function as an interface between brain and mind, between sleep and wake, and between unconsciousness and consciousness. This capacity for dreaming to provide a window between mind and brain was developed by Rene Descartes at the dawn of modern science. In his journal, dated November 10, 1619, he notes the ideas that came to him in a series of dreams:

> And finally, taking into account the fact that the same thoughts we have when we are awake can also come to us when asleep, without any of the later thoughts being true, I resolved to pretend that everything that had ever entered my mind was no more true than the illusions of my dream. For how does one know that the thoughts that come to us in our dreams are more false than the others, given that they are no less vivid or expressed?...our dreams ... represent to us various objects in the same way as our exterior senses do...what truth there is in them (our thoughts) ought infallibly to be found in those we have when awake rather than those we have in our dreams.[40]

This is Descartes' argument for the principle of Cartesian doubt—the willful suspension of all interpretations of experience that cannot be proved. Scientific methodology could be applied to waking reality and not to the improvable events of dream. From this perspective, dream is all that we cannot scientifically understand.[41] This dichotomy of mind/body has been codified and built into the structures of our fields of knowledge, a border dividing subjective from objective, conscious thought from nonconscious brain activity, science from art, and medicine from psychiatry. Philosophers have described this mind/brain border as the homogeneity constraint—that which prevents us from moving from between the subjective and the objective. Philosophically, we are locked into whichever side of the subjective—objective divide from which we start, a methodological obstacle that makes it seemingly impossible to cram the subjective and the objective into the same inferential space.[42] It was Sigmund Freud's contention that dreams could provide an interface into the psychodynamics and functioning of the mind. This worldview is often construed as being filled with the magic of the unconscious, a world in which the individual is not fully present or in volitional control, enveloped by dream just as a child is enveloped by his own world. The subject does not see where a dream is leading, yet she or he follows. We can use the dream information provided at this interface to alter our waking behavior, choose our relationships, make our decisions, and create waking products and activities based at least in part on our dreams.[43] In our art we create simulacrums of our dreams. Our consciousness is, in turn, altered at the interface by the interactions we have with our dreams.

The dream interface is bidirectional and multiplex, an interface at which we tap the same interior psychic confusion and dramatically ambivalent understanding of ourselves that we see reflected in a mirror. As in watching a film, we are in a dynamic as interactive spectators where the apparent mirror leads us to believe that we are present and involved with the images on the screen.[42] In viewing the dream (the interface), we are both enmeshed and displaced from ourselves, extending this identification into entertainment, product, and political marketing, and into our personal, social, and political lives. This interface is filled with our thoughts, our emotions, our memories, and our hopes, and as far more than a reflection, they come back to us.

For the computer gamer, spending significant amounts of waking time interacting with today's limited interfaces, the quality of sleep, dream content, and patterns of thought are altered.[32,39] When sleeping, many of us will dream of our experiences at the interface. New interface approaches will augment this access to the cognitive and physiologic systems utilized in sleep and dream states. This interface of dream is very likely to be bidirectional, shared, and subject to only limited volitional control. At times it may be a unique, bizarre, and hallucinatory experience tied to interactive processes or emotion and creativity. No dreamer experiencing such an interface, human or machine, is likely to ever experience their reality in quite the same way.

This is not the first time that changes in technology have induced a basic change in the way that we interface with the exterior world. Theatre audiences went rushing from the room when confronted with the first moving images of an onrushing train.[44] And cogent to this argument for the importance of dreaming as an interactive interface, black-and-white television influenced an entire generation to believe that their typical dreams were experienced in black and white.[45] We now sit quietly before an onrushing train. Vivid color and digital clarity have returned to our dreams. Altered and augmented by our experience at the interface, we continue to change.

## Notes

1. Nagel, T. (1994). Consciousness and objective reality. In R. Warner & T. Szubka (Eds.), *The mind-body problem*. Oxford: Blackwell. A wonderful quote from one of our finest philosophers.
2. Raskin, J. (2000). *The humane interface: New directions for designing interactive systems* (p. 10). Reading, MA: Addison-Wesley.
3. Barrs, B. (1998). *A cognitive theory of consciousness*. Cambridge: Cambridge University Press. The Global Platform concept for has slowly developed to become the primary construct utilized in attempts to cognitively and biologically understand the process of consciousness.
4. Vernon, D. (2005). Can neurofeedback training enhance performance? An evaluation of the evidence with implications for future research. *Applied Psychophysiology and Biofeedback, 30,* 165–205.
5. Ogheneovo, E. (2014). Software dysfunction: Why do software fail? *Journal of Computers and Communications, 2,* 25–35.
6. Raskin, J. (2000). *The humane interface: New directions for designing interactive systems* (p. 43). Reading, MA: Addison-Wesley.
7. Konvalinka, I., Bauer, M., Stahlhut, C., Hansen, C. K., Roepstorff, A., & Frith, C. D. (2005). Frontal alpha oscillations distinguish leaders from followers: Multivariate decoding of mutually interactive brains. *Neuroimage, 94,* 79–88.
8. Kurzwell, R. (2012). *How to create a mind: The secret of human thought revealed* (p. 72). New York: Penguin.
9. Hoskovek, J. (1966). Hypnopedia in the Soviet Union: A critical review of recent major experiments. *International Journal of Clinical and Experimental Hypnosis, 14,* 305–315.
10. Berger, R. (1963). Experimental modification of dream content by meaningful verbal stimuli. *British Journal of Psychiatry, 109,* 722–740.
11. Dement, W., & Wolpert, E. (1958). The relation of eye movements, body motility, and external stimuli to dream content. *Journal of Experimental Psychology, 55,* 543–553.
12. First look: How the Google glass UI really works. *Co.Design.* www.fastcodesign.com/1672314/first-look-how-the-google-glass-ui-really-works Accessed 03.08.16.
13. Selker, T. (2004). Visual attentive interfaces. *BT Technology Journal, 22,* 4.
14. Horsager, A., & Fine, L. (2016). The perceptual effects of chronic retinal stimulation. In G. Dagnelle (Ed.), *Visual prosthetics: Physiology, bioengineering, rehabilitation* (pp. 271–301). New York: Springer.
15. Wolpaw, J. R., Birbaumer, N., Heetderks, W. J., McFarland, D. J., Peckham, P. H., Schalk, G., et al. (2000). Brain-computer interface technology: A review of the first international meeting. *IEEE Transactions on Rehabilitation Engineering, 8*(2), 164–173.
16. Nicolelis, M., & Chapin, J. (2002). Controlling robots with mind. *Scientific American, 287*(4), 46–53.

17. Donchin, E., Spencer, K. M., & Wijesinghe, R. (2000). The mental prosthesis: Assessing the speed of a P300-based brain-computer interface. *IEEE Transactions on Rehabilitation Engineering, 8*(2), 174—179.
18. Spencer, K. M., Dien, J., & Donchin, E. (2001). Spatiotemporal analysis of the late ERP responses to deviant stimuli. *Psychophysiology, 38*(2), 343—358.
19. Babiloni, R., Cincotti, P., Lazzarini, L., Millan, J., Mouriiio, J., Varsta, M., et al. (2000). Linear classification of low-resolution EEG patterns produced by imagined hand movements. *IEEE Transactions on Rehabilitation Engineering, 8*(2), 186—188.
20. Farwell, L. A., & Donchin, E. (1988). Talking off the top of your head: Toward a mental prosthesis utilizing event-related brain potentials. *Electroencephalography and Clinical Neurophysiology, 70*(6), 510—523.
21. Buzsaki, G. (2006). *Rhythms of the brain.* Oxford: Oxford University Press.
22. Palaniappan, R. (2006). Utilizing gamma band to improve mental task based brain-computer interface design. *IEEE Transactions on Neural Systems and Rehabilitation Engineering, 14,* 299—303.
23. Cardin, J. A., Carlen, M., Meletis, K., Knoblich, U., Zhang, F., Deisseroth, K., et al. (2009). Driving fast-spiking cells induces gamma rhythm and controls sensory responses. *Nature, 459,* 663—667.
24. Pagel, J. F. (2012). The synchronous electrophysiology of conscious states. *Dreaming, 22,* 173—191. A detailed analysis of the proven and potential functioning capacities for this important CNS system.
25. Herrmann, W. M., & Schaerer, E. (1986). Pharmaco-EEG: Computer EEG analysis to describe the projection of drug effects on a functional cerebral level in humans. In F. H. Lopes da Silva, W. S. van Leeuwen, & A. Rémond (Eds.), *Clinical application of computer analysis of EEG and other neurophysiological signals, EEG handbook (revised series)* (Vol. 2, pp. 385—445). Amsterdam: Elsevier; Pagel, J. F. (1993). Modeling drug actions on electrophysiologic effects produced by EEG modulated potentials. *Human Psychopharmachology, 8,* 211—216.
26. Fell, J., Axmacher, N., & Haupt, S. (2010). From alpha to gamma: Electrophysiological correlates of meditation-related states of consciousness. *Medical Hypotheses, 75,* 218—224.
27. Lock, T. (1995). Stimulus dosing. In C. Freeman (Ed.), *The ECT handbook* (pp. 72—87). London: Royal College of Psychiatrists. This book is a window into what has been maintained from another era of psychiatry.
28. Cacioppo, J. T., Tassinary, L. G., & Berntson, G. G. (Eds.). (2007). *Handbook of psychophysiology* (3rd ed., p. 121). New York: Cambridge University Press.
29. Pascual-Leone, A., Davey, N., Rothwell, J., Wassermann, E. M., & Puri, B. K. (2002). *Handbook of transcranial magnetic stimulation.* London: Edward Arnold.
30. Jacobs, G. D., & Friedman, R. (2004). EEG spectral analysis of relaxation techniques. *Applied Psychophysiology and Biofeedback, 29,* 245—254.
31. Linden, M. T., & Radojevich, V. (1996). A controlled study of the effects of EEG biofeedback on cognition and behavior of children with attention deficit disorder and learning disabilities. *Biofeedback and Self-Regulation, 21,* 35—49.
32. Cho, B., Lee, J., Ku, J., Jang, D., Kim, J., Kim, I., et al. (2002). Attention enhancement system using virtual reality and EEG biofeedback. In *Proceedings of the IEEE Virtual Reality* (pp. 156—163). Los Alamitos, CA: IEEE Computer Society Press.
33. Lehmann, D., Faber, P., Achermann, P., Jeanmonod, D., Gianotti, L., & Pizzagalli, D. (2001). Brain sources of EEG gamma frequency during volitionally meditation-induced, altered states of consciousness, and experience of the self. *Psychiatry Research, 108,* 111—121.
34. Olgivie, R., Hunt, H., Tyson, P., Lucescu, M., & Jeankin, D. (1978). Searching for lucid dreams. *Sleep Research, 7,* 165.

35. Pagel, J. F. (2013). Lucid dreaming as sleep offset waking. *Sleep, 34*, Abstract suppl.; Holzinger, B., LaBerge, S., & Levitan, L. (2006). Psychophysiological correlates of lucid dreaming. *Dreaming, 16*, 88–95; Voss, U., Holzmann, R., Tuin, I., & Hobson, J. A. (2009). Lucid dreaming: A state of consciousness with features of both waking and non-lucid dreaming. *Sleep, 32*, 1191–1200.
36. Oak Ridge Associated Universities Panel for the Committee on Interagency Radiation Research and Policy Commission. (1992). *Health effects of low-frequency electric and magnetic fields*. Washington, DC: Oak Ridge Associated Universities (US Government). This book, as well, is reflective of another era, and the worries that persist particularly as to high-voltage power line environmental exposure.
37. Headrick, J. M. (1990). Looking over the horizon (HF radar). *IEEE Spectrum, 27*, 36–39; Garcia, C. (Director). (2015). *The Russian Woodpecker*. www.ioncinema.com/reviews/the-russian-woodpecker-review Assessed 20.10.16.
38. *The Russian Woodpecker—SETI@home*. https://setiathome.berkeley.edu/forum_thread.php?id = 79511 Assessed 20.10.16.
39. Gackenback, J., & Kurville, B. (2013). Cognitive structure associated with the lucid features of gamer's dreams. *Dreaming, 23*, 256–267. Gamers are our modern-day cyborg guinea pigs. Descartes, R. (1641). Objections against the meditations and replies. In J. M. Adler (Ed-in chief), *Great books of the Western world: Bacon, Spinoza and Descartes (1993)* (pp. 17, 21). Chicago, IL: Encyclopedia Britannica Inc.
40. Descartes, R. (1980). *Discourse on method* (D. A. Cress, Trans.). Indianapolis, IN: Hackett Publishing Co (Original work published 1637).
41. Flanagan, O. (1992). *Consciousness reconsidered* (p. 116). Cambridge, MA: MIT Press.
42. Lacan, J. (1979). The imaginary signifier. In *Four fundamental concepts of psychoanalysis* (A. Sheridan, Trans.). Harmondsworth: Penguin Books Ltd.
43. Pagel, J. F., & Vann, B. (1992). The effects of dreaming on awake behavior. *Dreaming, 2*(4), 229–237.
44. Lumiere Brothers. (1895). L'arrivée d'un train en gare de La Ciotat. In *Early cinema: Primitives and pioneers (1895–1910)*. London: BFI Video Publishing.
45. Schredl, M., Fuchedzhieva, A., Hämig, H., & Schindele, V. (2008). Do we think dreams are in black and white due to memory problems? *Dreaming, 18*, 175–180.

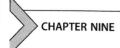

# CHAPTER NINE

# Interpreting the AI Dream

*Sometimes the machine's answer is as hallucinatory and imprecise as any bio-logically produced and interactively psychoanalyzed dream.*

**Pagel (2016)**

*A dream which is not interpreted is like a letter which is not read*
**Berakhot Talmud (approx. 500 BCE).[1]**

Dreams exist on the interface of sleeping consciousness. The dream is most apparent on awakening, on our reentry into waking consciousness. At that point, the dream provides cognitive feedback as to what has taken place in the brain during sleep. The dream can provide feedback on overall CNS status—positive or negative mood, varying degrees of disarray, as well as identifying areas of overall concern. The recall of the interface (dream) is affected by a series of well-described variables (see Chapter 1: Dreaming: The Human Perspective). It is at this point that each dreamer confronts the experienced dream. The dreamer applies to the dream a language, a cognitive organization, a narrative structure, judgment, and any requirements for shared presentation. This is interpretation. In a biologic system, this process of dream recall followed by interpretation is the point or level of interface at which digital on—off signals (neuron firing or not firing in a biological system) are converted into an analogue description of the cognitive processing of an otherwise interior digital world. Such analogues are metaphors. Such metaphors are dreams.

In basic format, all neural and computer processing is digital. In computer systems, binary (01010101) coded information is incorporated into electronic bits stored either in the local memory system of the computer or in a remote memory system, such as the Cloud/Internet. In biologic nervous systems, the on—off process is determined and delineated in nerve cells (neurons) that either fire (conducting a signal) or do not fire, in response to impinging input. Such an on—off process can be viewed, as well, as a binary process. Both the human brain and the digitally programmed computer can be seen as different instantiations of the same kind of device, generating intelligent behaviors by manipulating symbols

*Machine Dreaming and Consciousness.*
DOI: http://dx.doi.org/10.1016/B978-0-12-803720-1.00009-8

with formal rules.[2] On the input side, this digital coding is cognitively integrated to provide a representation of externally experienced reality. This representation is one of many possible ways to describe exterior reality. The addition of a time marker to two-dimensional digital coding produces a virtual three-dimensional framework that can be utilized to represent our relationship and/or the computer's relationship to external space. Sufficiently complex and broadly implemented machines can incorporate multidimensional sensory array information into data histories that approach the complexity of the human memory experience.

At the input interface exterior reality is encoded as a digital metaphor. Due to the limits of "simple" on−off coding and the constrained set of sensors use to describe the exterior environment as three-dimensional space, much of the actual nature of reality is lost at the interface. Neither we humans, nor computers, can "see" much of what is taking place in the exterior world. That impinging world is constructed of different energies (e.g., electromagnetic wavelengths and energy types), different spatial structures (e.g., other dimensions), and different sensory modalities (e.g., quantum probability, empty space) from those that either we or our machine creations have the capacity to represent and examine. The most important characteristic required for the creation of a digital representation of the exterior world is that the representation has consistency. Any schema that we use must produce a consistent representation of the exterior environment so that we can use that information to rationally interact with the surrounding world.

Within the human CNS, visual digital sensory data are topographically represented, presented, and displayed on networks of neurons much like pixels are displayed on a television screen. Like pixels, these representations are not fully digital—they do not provide a concrete one-on-one representation, or numeric specificity. They are not fully analogue, meaning that beyond visual representation they can be mathematically analyzed and incorporated into biologic digital memory systems. Analysis and data integration is then accomplished through neural networks, and other forms of memory incorporation, that are then available for tertiary cognitive processing.

In machines, attempts are being made to parody human representational systems.[3] In current machine systems, this representation is most often mathematical, based on the use of calculus and Fourier transforms to develop statistical descriptions of data that can be analyzed, or visually projected through the transference of pixel-based data onto recording media such as film or laser-recorded discs. Both approaches, biologic and machine, allow for a level of intermediate and internal data presentation that approximates the exterior world. These data, presented in an apparently analogue manner, can then be mathematically and/or neurologically processed. The results of that processing can then be utilized for cognitive interaction, not just for assessment, but also at the level of output, when the products of such analysis enter shared consciousness and social interaction.

The out-point of the digital/analogue interface is at the point of data presentation in the machine, and on awakening and during waking in the human. It is at this point that interpretation, assessment, and integration of data takes place. Machine-based data, when presented as a set of numbers or pixels, is digitally derivative. Even then, the requirement for human interpretation means that data are always analyzed by the interpreting human in an analogue and metaphoric manner. The data presented at that machine interface (the dream in a biologic system) are a cognitive response to an analogue experience that took place earlier during waking and was then digitally incorporated into a memory system.

## DREAM INTERPRETATION

It was Freud's insight that a manifest (presented) dream could be interpreted and analyzed, and that this presented report could be utilized to understand an analysand's psychodynamic process.[4] For a trained psychoanalyst, the personal dynamics of the dream report could then be approached on different levels: familial and parental relationships, belief systems and taboos, patterns of psychiatric illness, and perceived or experienced trauma, as well as on the shared levels of a collective unconscious built on myths and symbols. While psychoanalysis is used now infrequently as a psychiatric diagnostic and therapeutic approach, it remains as a primary structured approach utilized in the attempt to understand the psychological basis and the potential origin of psychiatric illness. It remains a dominant approach in art and film analysis and criticism, and is still utilized in attempts towards individual self-understanding.[5]

In dream content analysis, psychoanalysis remains a predominate force. Psychoanalytic-based transference and expectations continue to cloud and confuse the results of studies. Currently, dream researchers utilize computer-assisted dream content analysis in an attempt to achieve the consistent and reproducible results that were lacking in the anecdotal research of the psychoanalytic era.[6] The results attained in such studies have been somewhat disappointing, particularly for psychoanalytically based practitioners. The only provable correlates in such tightly controlled studies have been gender differences and the continuity of dream content with waking experience. In these studies, as postulated by psychoanalytic theorists, depressed individuals are more likely to have depressing and negative dream content. However, that content is part of the psychodynamics of their illness only in that it resembles and reflects their waking thought. Anxious individuals are more likely to have confused and anxiety-ridden dream content. Schizophrenics are more likely to have thought disordered, unusual, and bizarre dreaming.[7] There is little evidence to suggest that the psychodynamic patterns apparent in these individual's reported dreams is somehow the cause or origin of their illnesses. That association is more likely to be found in the individual on the other side of the psychotherapeutic interface—in the beliefs, training, and preconceptions of the dream interpreter. Outside continuity, in controlled studies, gender is the only other characteristic consistently affecting dream content. If a study does not demonstrate a statistically significant gender difference, there is likely a methodological problem in that study. The data are likely to somehow be corrupted.[8]

## MACHINE DATA PRESENTATION

Computer data can be reported as basic binary on—off (010101) telemetry. More often, AI data are presented as numbers, words, or images. In Internet system design, artificial neural network construction, and in statistical analysis, for each level of increased complexity variables are added that can alter the presented results so that dysfunction becomes more probable as the complexity increases. Increasingly complex processing can produce a significant proportion of outcomes that can be considered as indeterminate or hallucinatory. As noted previously, an alternative and apparently real version of reality is produced in three of the eight results obtained based on the basic hardware structure of neural network processing. Flexible, less-controlled, and probability-based programming languages increase the likelihood for such indeterminate outcomes.

Humans are visual creatures. The visual projection of results is often desired. A visual presentation of results can appear to be more intuitive and meaningful. The results of complex analytic evaluations, such as weather change over time, are almost impossible to evaluate when presented numerically. Once the decision is made to visually present results, it becomes far more difficult to mathematically compare and evaluate the results. This is particularly true for those results that are changing over time, as in the case of the filmatic presentation of climate change. The results of such complex analytic paradigms can be unique and nonrepeatable, even when the same initial data input and processing protocols are applied. These results can be construed as evidence for machine dysfunction, hypothetical and nonapplicable to real-world situations. When the obtained results vary, it is only those results that are seemingly consistent with expected outcomes, the researchers' beliefs, or the presenter's aesthetic, that are likely to be utilized. Yet, indeterminate and hallucinatory results from such analyses can be used to produce remarkably diffuse and vivid imagery. Google personnel call such images "computer-generated dreams."[9]

Minimally controlled and recurrently stacked self-learning neural networks when used to analyze speech and language will develop a high-dimensional feature space for each word. Words and signs (tokens) with similar representations will have similar representations in this high-definition space. Computer instructions and data in memory are also tokens. AI data can be tokenized at levels of abstraction varying form the single data point to the overall state of a neural network. Each token, represented as a single symbol, can be integrated and implemented in parallel to produce the information available for final interpretation. In this computer-derived space, a dimension sometimes develops that correlates with gender independent of the specific word meaning. Gender difference is a basic and consistent characteristic of such analyses, just as in studies used to analyze the content of dreams.[10] It is interesting that as in dream content research, the finding of a consistent gender variation may correlate with the methodological objectivity of the study.

## MACHINE DATA INTERPRETATION

At the point of download and integration into focused waking consciousness, tokenized dream and data reports have the requirement of human interpretation. At this point interface problems and variables come into play. These include some of the same variables that have affected human attempts to psychodynamically understand their own dreams and behaviors. Expectations, beliefs, transference, and conscious manipulation typify the human approach to any data, result, or reported dream. Science, in its most basic aspect, is a belief system, even if it is one designed to be based on testable experiments and repeatable hypotheses. The computer at its most basic level, functions as the calculator of Lebienz, as the scientist's extender. For some "scientists" the computer's greatest use is in data mining and statistical manipulation. The nonscientist without even these constraints, may search only for data and/or images that support a personal pattern of belief, politics, religious or sexual orientation, entertainment, and/or desire. At the machine interface, presented data enter this human world of analogy and metaphor, interpreted and analyzed in what (for the machine) is an appallingly nonintelligent and nonprecise manner.

At the point of download, the data report requires human interpretation. Interface problems and variables as well as human transference, belief systems, expectations, and even intentional attempts at fraud can alter the interpretation of results. At this machine output interface, presented data enter the human world of analogy and metaphor in which the data are spun, interpreted, and analyzed to produce a metaphoric, analogous, and analogue perspective of the universe. The answer produced is most often goal-reflective, having continuity with the problem presented. But sometimes the machine's answer is as hallucinatory and imprecise as any biologically produced and interactively psychoanalyzed dream. These answers can present a potentially useful alternative view of the problem presented, and the system's experience of its own external reality. Systems are often programmed to discard, ignore, or deemphasize results that are inconsistent or out of the range of goals set by the programmer. Such results are often considered to be evidence for machine dysfunction, and particularly when the obtained results vary markedly, the only results utilized will be those consistent with expected outcomes, the researchers' beliefs, or the presenter's aesthetic.

The human—computer interface interaction taking place at output, is much like the dream presented for interpretation on waking. Environment interaction at input, is processed with nonconscious digital coding to produce a metaphoric, analogous, and analogue perspective of the universe. The human dream is an experience that can mimic all human senses and sensibilities. To dream is to experience that which one can perceive as stimulus via a nonsensory path, the objects, and actions of experience. The dream reflects, and has continuity, but is not tightly correlated with that exterior existence. The data analysis presented by an AI system, if based on a sufficiently complex instillation of data and processing, can require for that analysis the full extent of the machine's sensory and cognitive capacity, and at least a portion of the available memory stores. The answer produced most often reflects and has continuity with the question asked. But that is not always true. Sometimes the machine's answer is as hallucinatory and imprecise as any biologically produced dream—a strangely structured, somewhat askew, often hard to remember, altered, and yet potentially useful alternative view of external experience and reality.

## Notes

1. Frieden, K. (1993). Talmudic dream interpretation, Freudian ambivalence, deconstruction. Statement attributed to Rabbi Chisda. In C. Ruppercht (Ed.), *The dream and the text: Essays on literature and language* (p. 104). Albany, NY: State University of New York Press.
2. Newell, A., & Simon, H. (1976). Computer science as empirical enquiry: Symbols and search. *Communications of the ACM, 19,* 113–126; Dreyfus, H., & Dreyfus, S. (1988). Making a mind versus modeling the brain: Artificial intelligence back at a branchpoint. *Artificial Intelligence, 117,* 15–43.
3. Parasi, D. (2007). Mental robotics. In A. Chella & R. Manzotti (Eds.), *Artificial consciousness* (pp. 191–211). Charlottesville, VA: Imprint Academic.
4. Freud, S. (1953). The interpretation of dreams. In S. James (Ed.), *The standard editions of the complete psychological works of Sigmund Freud* (Vols. IV and V). London: Hogarth Press.
5. Pagel, J. F. (2014). *Dream science: Exploring the forms of consciousness.* Oxford: Academic Press (Elsevier).
6. Domhoff, G. W. (2003). *The scientific study of dreams: Neural networks, cognitive development, and content analysis.* Washington, DC: American Psychological Association.
7. Yu, C. (2014). Normality, pathology, and dreaming. *Dreaming, 24,* 203–216.
8. Kramer, M. (2007). *The dream experience: A system exploration.* New York: Routledge.
9. Google's AI can dream, and here's what it looks like. *IFLScience.* www.iflscience.com/technology/artificial-intelligence-dream Accessed 13.09.16.
10. Wood, M. (2016). The concept of "cat face": Paul Taylor on machine learning. *London Review of Books, 38*(16), 30–32.

# CHAPTER TEN

# Creating the Perfect Zombie

*They were able to pack over ten billion neuristor-type cells into a very small area—around a cubic foot. They aimed for that magic figure because that is approximately the number of nerve cells in the human brain. That is what I meant when I said that it wasn't really a computer. They were actually working in the area of artificial intelligence, no matter what they called it.*

**Zelanzy R. (1976) My Name is Legion.[1]**

Computers, as originally conceived, were designed to manipulate bits of digital data presented symbolically as numbers. The role of the computer programmer was to manipulate these symbols by using a set of formal rules developed from the fields of mathematics and the formal logics of philosophy. Some hoped that artificial intelligence (AI) might develop, based on the manipulation of a physical signal system that could provide "the necessary and sufficient means for general intelligent action."[2]

Scientific theory and procedure has a long history in Western philosophy and science, dating back to Plato and Aristotle. Descartes, Hobbs, Leibniz, and Kant all approached science and philosophy as a search for underlying rules, logics, and formulas—a search for the basic simples and symbols defining our external and internal existence. The scientific approach was intrinsic to developing 20th century empiric philosophy. Husserl postulated that the world, as humans view it, is a complex system of facts, correlated by beliefs, modified by conditions of truth called validities.[3] Ludwig Wittgenstein in his Tratatus Logico—Philosophieus built the following argument:

1. The world is the totality of facts, not of things;
2. An atomic fact is a combination of arguments;
3. If all objects are given, then thereby all facts are given;
4. We make to ourselves pictures of facts;
5. The elements of the picture are combined with one another in a definite way, represents that the things are combined with one another.[4]

In the 20th century, using such a logic, many philosophers and most neuroscientists adopted the perspective of naturalism—the belief that all nonphysical properties are either reducible to or must be realized or

*Machine Dreaming and Consciousness.*
DOI: http://dx.doi.org/10.1016/B978-0-12-803720-1.00010-4

implemented in physical properties. As based on this philosophic construct, AI is an attempt to logically structure in an artificial system the various primitive elements and their relationships that make up the world, in a way that parodies human functioning in the same construct.[5]

At the dawn of the computing era, this basic philosophic perspective led many in the field to think that controlled symbolic information-processing in the new computing format would quickly lead to strong AI—machines as intelligent or more intelligent than humans. Fairly quickly, it was demonstrated that computer systems could function as general problem solvers, utilizing the process of search, means, and analysis to perform better than humans in set attempts to attain described goals. Extending this accomplishment, AI systems were developed that could function on a human or super-human level within areas or domains with clearly circumscribed facts and rules. Systems were designed to be able to function at super-human levels in games playing roles such as in chess competitions, and in environments with set constraints (e.g., space exploration). Both of these approaches, sometimes described as cognitive simulation and microworlds, have turned out to be successful and attainable applications for AI.[6]

Today, however, the limitations of parametrically controlled computer systems have become particularly obvious. This is especially true in the field of robotics—independently functioning AI. What humans construe as everyday know-how—how to move in space, how not to fall over, how to procedurally determine the next appropriate step in a changing environment—has been extraordinarily difficult to program or reduce into a set operative protocol of facts and rules. From the programming perspective, the commonsense world in which we as humans live and operate has turned out to be a world that is sometimes based only minimally on logic and theoretic structure. The human child plays with forms, fluids, and solids for years in order to develop typical skilled responses to their typical behavior in typical circumstances, developing these skills in the midst of socially important interactional constructs in order to develop the required background understanding required for functioning in our commonsense world.[7]

Both Heidegger and Wittgenstein, confronted philosophically with the limitations of logical formulations, have suggested that humans function in the real world without any formal theory of mind, behaving intelligently in this world without having any theory of the world. Wittgenstein rejected his own earlier work in suggesting that there are no actual unconstrained facts, no absolute metaphors in which facts exist free of context and purpose.[8] Heidegger suggested that there is no way to formally represent the exterior world with a set of facts and their set relationships.[9] Humans are evidently able to function intelligently in the world without having a theory or a set of rules and logics for behaving in that world. This philosophical bombshell fell into an AI community frustrated by the limitations of traditional goal-oriented and physical-symbol programming approaches to computer processing. In order to design systems that could function in the commonsense human world, programming required that there be a set of logics that governed both human and machine behavior. If such was not true, and the actions of our conscious minds were nonalgorithmic, the world as we experience was likely to be both deterministic and noncomputable.[10] This became a major philosophical and operational conundrum for AI programmers, limiting their ability to develop AI systems able to function in a routine, commonsense-based, human world rarely based on set relationships and logics.

## NEURAL NETS

In the last half of the 20th century, it became generally accepted that the aspects of brain functioning (mind) occurred secondary to underlying brain activity. Using brain slice studies, fMRI, PET, SQUIB, and micropipette techniques, neuroscientists described the neuroanatomical, neurochemical, electrophysiological, and neuropsychatiric characteristics of the brain, presenting much of this work as research into brain cognitive function (mind). Real-time scanning was used to document particular areas of the brain active when an individual is asked to think of a mind-based concept such as God (or art, or politics, or love).[10] Conclusions seemed to logically follow:

1. Humans who utilize a similar neuroanatomic area are also thinking of God;
2. Since this area is present in our CNS, it is a human characteristic to think of God;
3. Since we have such a neuroanatomic area, this is evidence that we share the requirement for God;
4. Such a shared neuroanatomic area is evidence for the existence of God; and

**5.** Since animals have similar activity in similar areas of their CNS, they are also thinking of God.[11]

This and similar logic series have been religiously proselytized.[12] Such "evidence-based" neuroanatomic (brain = mind) perspectives and theories were then used to support the wide spectrum of neuroconsciousness theories suggesting that a concrete, neuroanatomic correlation existed between brain activity and mind function. Once adopted, this perspective led logically to the possibility that an artificially created neural system might also have the capacity to approximate the functions and processes of mind.

Artificially created neural-net systems provide an option to the algorithmic or parametric physical symbol programming utilized by most current computer systems that have had such difficulty in approximating human patterns of commonsense behavior.[13] Potentially, the more flexible and less-controlled neural-net systems would have the capacity for approximating commonsense human behaviors. Such systems might develop a capacity for intelligent behavior without requiring the creator of such a system to have either a theoretic explanation or an understanding of the logical construct producing such behavior.

## CREATING THE PERFECT ZOMBIE

It is within our technical capacity to create that which we do not necessarily understand. We can now artificially create at least a portion of the physical properties and systems of the human CNS. Artificial neural-net systems, recreated on a micro- and macrofeature level, can be incorporated into structured multilayer systems reflecting current concepts of CNS operative functioning. These systems can be designed to function independently, without requiring symbolic information-processing and programming controls. This approach avoids any requirement that either the programmer or the machine have a theory or understanding of the exterior world, or the interior processes required for functioning in that world.

Advances in technology have repeatedly left scientists in similar positions. The genetic sequencing of the human genome, an obvious technical triumph, is a clear example. Despite abundant self-congratulatory publicity, our very limited understanding of genetic process and function has severely limited the expected advances based on this remarkable advance in technology. The social benefits that have been derived from genetic sequencing have rarely been medical or life-saving. Genetic sequencing is used instead as a method of personal identification—a forensic extension of fingerprinting. While this use of genetic coding is socially important, it is an impressively limited use of this basic biologic control code utilized in evolution, development, cellular functioning, all levels of physiology, and as a template for consciousness. The hoped-for expansions in the diagnosis and treatment of disease and behavior have been, to this point, quite limited. True breakthroughs are yet to be realized.

The sequencing of the genome does, however, provide a basic template on which to build other, even more complex systems, that we do not yet understand. The human CNS is composed of 100 billion neurons connected by 100 trillion synapses, each individually controlled by 80,000 genes (3 billion basepairs) affected and interconnected by multiple electrical, ionic, energy, and chemical systems that exert their effects inside and outside neural pathways. Despite such a level of extreme complexity, the creation of an equivalent artificial system is within the realm of technical possibility.[14] Starting at the level of genetic coding, simulacrums of the CNS are now being constructed.

## NEUROANATOMIC ZOMBIES

Biologically derivative neural-net development has focused on the micro- and macroneuroanatomy of the brain. From the gross perspective, the brain is subdivided into various pathologically and anatomically differentiated parts (brain stem, cortex, cerebellum, etc.) that include approximately 100 subdivisions generally described as nuclei or loci specialized for various different sensory, cognitive, and motor functions. Each of these cortical areas is constructed of subunits, local groups, or pools of cells, that act in a coordinated way: columns, cell assemblies, microcircuits, or as networks of individual nerve cells each interconnected by axon and dendritic synaptic interfaces. Individual neurons interconnect with glial and other support cells form basic units of this anatomic system at their own microscopic level of scale. Each neuron is a consensually functioning organism (cell) that can be subdivided into compartments, synapses, channels, and molecules each with physiological and dynamical properties. Within and outside the cellular nucleus, the genomic systems of DNA and RNA are variably expressed in response to cellular messenger, protein, pH, ATP, electrolyte, and electrical frequency changes. Extending from the organ brain down to the level of DNA coding, the series of integrated levels in the mammal CNS have been postulated to include at least 17 levels of interactive complexity.[15]

Major attempts are currently underway to further analyze and then artificially create constructs of the mammalian CNS. At the Allen Institute in Seattle, neuroscientists have focused on the spatial mapping of CNS gene expression in the mouse. Techniques have been developed in which mouse CNS neural activity and gene expression can be monitored on a real-time basis using the technique of colorimetric in situ hybridization. Datasets with cellular-level spatial resolution are being used to produce cellular transcriptomic profiles of specific neuroanatomic regions in an attempt to further dissect and derive the molecular and genetic underpinnings of brain function.[16] Such genetic expression profiles offer the potential for elucidating the basic DNA programming patterns utilized in active functioning by the mammalian CNS.

The European Union has invested major research funds into an even more ambitious project, through the École Polytechnique Fédérale de Lausanne (EPFL). There, Henry Markram leads the attempt to design and produce a supercomputer based on multilevel neural network architecture. The initial goal of the project, the simulation of a rat neocortical column, considered by some researchers to be the smallest functional unit of the neocortex, was completed in 2006. In rats, each column is about 2 mm in length, has a diameter of 0.5 mm, containing approximately 10,000 neurons ($10^8$ synapses). The ultimate goal of this project is to allow for parallel simulation of large numbers of connected columns in order to reconstitute a whole neocortex (in humans about 1 million cortical columns).[17] At EPFL, the first-draft digital reconstruction of the microcircuitry of the somatosensory cortex of juvenile rat used cellular and synaptic organizing principles to algorithmically reconstruct detailed anatomy and physiology in a neocortical volume of $0.29 \pm 0.01$ mm$^3$ containing $\sim$31,000 neurons with 55 layer-specific morphological and 207 morpho-electrical neuron subtypes. This network of digitally reconstructed neurons included $\sim$8 million connections with $\sim$37 million synapses. Physiological electrical fields applied to this system produce a spectrum of network states that demonstrate a sharp transition from synchronous to asynchronous activity.[18] Markham has predicted that his laboratory will produce a system with complexity equivalent to the human CNS within the next 10 years.[15]

It is widely suspected that similar projects are underway utilizing governmental support in countries with far less transparency as to research status and results. Several countries have developed the technical capacity required for such research projects. China boasts the world's fastest supercomputers, including the Tianhe-2, built by China's National University of Defense Technology and housed at the National Super Computer Center in Guangzhou. One of its published uses is to be in the derivation and analysis of gene expression.[19]

The human CNS is among the most complex of systems that we have attempted to understand. Such cognitive systems are large, multiscale, nonlinear, highly heterogeneous, and highly interactive. An artificial system built on this model is an ideal construct for testing theories postulating that highly integrated complexity can lead to the emergence of human-equivalent consciousness. Such zombie systems should approximate the level of anatomic complexity present in the human CNS. The collateral postulate is that the level of structural complexity, measured as simultaneous integration and segregation of activity during different cognitive processing states, should be a direct measure of the level of consciousness attained.[20] As based on this complexity = consciousness theory, the perfect zombie would have the capacity for attaining levels and types of consciousness equivalent to that attainable in the human.

## LIMITATIONS IN CREATING THE NEUROANATOMIC ZOMBIE: CNS COMPLEXITY

Despite the hopes and assertions surrounding these projects, the perfect zombie still exists as a creature of our imagination (Fig. 10.1). While approaches that incorporate genomic variability, artificial neurons, and structural layering are exceedingly complex, these approaches are based on attempts to recreate what we currently know or postulate of pathophysical neural anatomy. The spatial and temporal structure of the brain functions on a wide and intermingled range of scales. Known factors involved and affecting CNS neuron functioning include electrophysiologic, neurochemical, neuroglial, and neuroendocrine systems.[21] These complex systems function in concert as well as independently of neuroanatomic transmission-line interconnections. Other factors affecting overall CNS functioning include: individual variability, environment, social

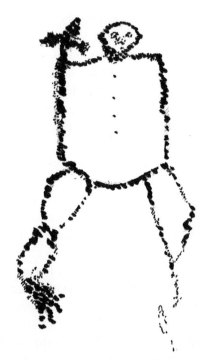

**Figure 10.1** The one-legged zombie—Mesa Pietra; Trail 2.

effects, belief system effects, as well as the spectrum of neurological and psychiatric illnesses. The neuroanatomic system of the CNS functions in environmental and temporal interaction. Temporally, the electrical, chemical, genetic, and endocrine dynamics of the brain span many orders of magnitude. Synaptic, magnetic, genetic, and electrical processes occur and alter within a submillisecond to millisecond range. Perceptual and thought processes happen in fractions of seconds to perhaps hours, and memory phenomena last for seconds to many years. Circadian and ultracircadian rhythms relate brain function to the external environment, including the effects of solar and lunar light and tidal cycles. Even slower processes affect the CNS on genetic, molecular, and evolutionary timescales. Each process, each CNS function, is embedded in a network of temporal and structural interactions and dependencies. Each biological system is also a physical system with the characteristics of a liquid, a gas, or a solid, each composed of an interactive atomic and subatomic structure. These inorganic factors affect and define the extent and characteristics of biological processes. These factors are likely to affect the manner and approaches that we utilize in our CNS to construct physically consistent representations of external and internal matter and space.

Beyond the known complexity of these systems, there is still much that is unknown about brain functioning. Neuroconsciousness theories suggesting direct correlates between mind and brain are clearly overly simplistic (e.g., REM sleep is not equivalent to dreaming, there is no on—off switch for sleep and/or consciousness, and there is no specifically located neural site for mind-based concepts such as God, love, and/or beauty). There is far more not known than there is known about CNS operation and functioning. Even what we think we know is debatable on many levels, and much is likely incorrect. By example, in the last 10 years as real-time function-based brain scanning data have become available, it has become obvious that the areas of brain activation described by this scanning are quite often not the same areas of brain neuroanatomy, neural transmission line tracts, and control nuclei that were described in earlier pathological studies. Scans indicate that neural activity associated with particular brain functions is often diffuse, in widely separated areas of the brain, and often in areas not previously suspected based on pathologic data to have roles in those functions. Functional scanning indicates, as well, that specific areas of the CNS may be deactivated rather than activated in association with specific functions. This lack or suppression of CNS activity in certain areas also alters brain functioning, sometimes in cognitively useful ways.[22] That is not to say that consistent patterns in data suggesting brain/mind correlates are incorrect, but rather to indicate that such patterns are incomplete, affected by the perspective and bias of theorists and researchers, and developed without a clear understanding of CNS operation and process. The 17 levels of neuroanatomic neural-net interactions describe but one level of the complex process of cognition. Current neuroanotomic zombie approaches are addressing only a subset of what is known. And what we know of CNS functioning is changing rapidly.

## PERFECT ZOMBIES

If anything resembling the human CNS is to be created as a functional system, more than the technical creation of anatomy equivalents will be required. A perfect zombie will need to incorporate the other known and unknown systems required for human CNS functioning. The neuroscientists involved in the zombie projects have approached complex systems such as electrophysiology and neurochemistry as background systems for the neuroanatomy that can be parodied by putting the system in a chemical bath, or by using set electrical shocks. The current knowledge base and known complexity of these systems will have to be integrated with the neuroanatomic and genetic coding equivalents if anything approximating a perfect zombie is ever to be created. As noted repeatedly in this book, our understanding of the CNS is still quite limited. As these projects progress, additional physiologic systems required for CNS functioning are likely to be discovered.

Despite the limits of our understanding, we are proceeding rapidly into a future that will include artificial supercomputers structured on neuroanatomically based brain equivalents. The inventor Ray Kurzweil, now working at Google, has predicted that by 2020 there will be computers able to model the human brain, and by 2029 there will be neural-net-based systems able to run human-equivalent brain simulations.[23] We are embarking on this journey with a very limited understanding of the workings of our CNS and its relationship to consciousness. Humans have learned to function intelligently in this world without having a theory or a set of rules and logics for behavior. Machines created in our image will also need the ability to function independently of rules and logics. The question remains as to how well the zombies that we are creating will be able to function in this world. There is the possibility that such machines will have even less ability to function than our current symbolic logic supercomputers. There is also the possibility of "singularity"—a term that some are using to describe a machine that would possess a generalized superintelligence, and the capacity to solve problems, learn, and take effective human-like actions in a variety of environments.[24] A created, self-aware, self-improving system would likely have the basic human drives of efficiency, self-preservation, resource acquisition, and creativity. These drives would be developed in order to discern predictable problems, to achieve its goals.[25] Such a superintelligent system is likely to be able to proceed independently to define its world. Such a system, more intelligent than the human, might have the capacity to solve apparently insoluble problems. Cancer might be cured, life extended, and the laws of physics manipulated to allow for interstellar travel. That is the dream, in which dream is defined as wish fulfillment. Today there are many complex problems without apparent solutions. Consider human-initiated global warming. After the "singularity," a perfect zombie with no "conscious" or logical reason for human preservation might make the decision and have the capacity to eliminate the obvious perpetrator of that dysfunction. That is the nightmare.

## Notes

1. Zelanzy, R. (1976). *My name is Legion* (p. 150). New York: A Del Rey Book/ Ballantine. Some of the greatest of science fiction writers were clearly precognitive. This was not fiction.
2. Newell, A., & Simon, H. (1981). Computer science as empirical enquiry: Symbols and search. In J. Haugeland (Ed.), *Mind design* (p. 41). Cambridge, MA: MIT Press.
3. Husserl, E. (1970). *Crisis of European sciences and transcendental phenomenology* (D. Carr, Trans.). Evanston, IL: Northwestern University Press.
4. Wittgenstein, L. (1960). *Tratatus logico-philosophieus*. London: Routledge & Kegan Paul.
5. Cussins, A. (1990). The connectionist construction of concepts. In M. Boden (Ed.), *The philosophy of artificial intelligence* (pp. 368–440; reprint 2005). Oxford: Oxford University Press.
6. Franklin, S. (2014). History, motivations, and core themes. In K. Frankish & W. Ramsey (Eds.), *The Cambridge handbook of artificial intelligence* (pp. 15–33). Cambridge: Cambridge University Press.
7. Dreyfus, H., & Dreyfus, S. (1988). Making a mind versus modeling the brain: Artificial intelligence back at a branchpoint. *Artificial Intelligence*, 117(1), 15–43.
8. Wittgenstein, L. (1975). *Philosophical remarks*. Chicago, IL: University of Chicago.
9. Heidegger, M. (1962). *Being and time* (p. 121). New York: Harper & Row. For the machine, $2 + 2$ must always equal 4. For the human there is no evident requirement for the veracity of truth or fact, a finding emphasized recently in the political arena.
10. Penrose, R. (1989). *The emperor's new mind: Concerning computers, minds, and the laws of physics* (p. 220). London: Vintage.
11. Frank Krueger, K., Barbey, A., McCabe, K., Strenziok, M., Zamboni, G., Solomon, J., et al. (2009). Cognitive and neural foundations of religious belief. *PNAS*, *106*(12), 4876–4881; published ahead of print March 9, 2009. Available from http://dx.doi. org/10.1073/pnas.0811717106; Alper, M. (2008). *The "God" part of the brain: A scientific interpretation of human spirituality and God*. Naperville, IL: Sourcebooks Inc.
12. Wilfried, A. (2009). Neurotheology: What can we expect from a (future) catholic version? *Theology and Science*, 7, 163–174. Available from http://dx.doi.org/10.1080/ 14746700902796528.
13. Parasi, D. (2007). Mental robotics. In A. Chella & R. Manzotti (Eds.), *Artificial consciousness* (pp. 191–211). Charlottesville, VA: Imprint Academic.
14. Markham, H. (2009). *A brain in a supercomputer*. TEDGlobal. Filmed July 2009. This area of zombie systems is changing rapidly. Much data is also protected through patent law and governmental secrecy, so that the best data available for reference are from presentations and blogs.
15. Markham, H. (2014). *Toward a science of consciousness* (p. 117). Tucson, AZ: University of Arizona, Center for Consciousness Studies.
16. Sualin, S., & Hohmann, J. (2007). Insights from spatially mapped gene expression in the mouse brain. *Human Molecular Genetics*, *16*, R209–R219.
17. Graham-Rowe, D. (June 2005). Mission to build a simulated brain begins. *NewScientist*; Abbott, A. (2013). Billion-euro brain simulation and graphene projects win European funds. *Nature*, January 23.

18. Markham, H., Muller, E., Ramasuany, S., Reimann, M., Abdellah, M., Sanchez, C., et al. (2015). Reconstruction and simulation of neocortical microcircuitry. *Cell, 163,* 456−492.
19. Tiezzi, S. (2015). US to challenge China for world's fastest supercomputer. *The Diplomat.* thediplomat.com Accessed 27.02.16. (China has recently developed an even more complex faster system).
20. Tononi, G. (2004). An information integration theory of consciousness. *BMC Neuroscience, 5,* 42.
21. Pagel, J. F. (2014). *Dream science: Exploring the forms of consciousness.* Oxford: Academic Press (Elsevier).
22. Andrews-Hanna, J. (2011). The brain's default network and its adaptive role in internal mentation. *The Neuroscientist, 18,* 1−20.
23. Kurzweil, R. (2005). *The singularity is near, when humans transcend biology.* New York: Viking Press.
24. Barrat, J. (2013). *Our final invention: Artificial intelligence and the end of the human era* (pp. 214−215). New York: Thomas Dunne Books.
25. Omohundro, S. (2008). *The nature of self-improving artificial intelligence.* http://selfaware-systems.files.wordpress.com/2008/01/nature_of_self_improving_ai.pdf/.

# The Philosophy of Machine Dreaming

Dream science and AI can be approached without resorting to an inquisitive structured philosophic approach to analytic thought. But for this book, the intuitional framework of philosophy provides a coherent framework for topics as diverse as dream and computer science. The Ancient Greek philosophers built their structures of logic around attempts to understand the meaning and significance of dreams. In kick-starting the advance in Western thought that we now call the Enlightenment, Rene Descartes discovered a logic for scientific method in his dreams. He used the power of that argument to describe the differences between waking experience and dreaming. The dichotomy that he described, between the physical and the mental—between mind and brain—still bedevils us in our attempts to understand consciousness.

Computer programming is an approach to philosophic logic reduced to mathematical form. Every mathematical proposition and every function of propositional calculus can be factored utilizing the digital computing capacity of a Turing machine. And every function of a Turing machine can be computed using an artificial neural network.[1] The concept of AI, now central to the philosophy of cognitive science, has required that an entire epistemology be built around the scientific study of intelligence.[2] The need to delineate aspects of human and machine intelligence has pushed philosophers to develop precise understandings of cognitive topics as diverse as emotion, belief, intentionality, attention, and volition. The possibility of consciousness in AI systems has led to a deconstruction in the fields of consciousness study. Each discussant has defined the concept of consciousness differently, using logics and perspectives based on what are often very different epistemologies and experience. The ways that we conceive and view our computing systems is now how we look at the brain. Both the brain and AI systems manipulate formal symbols in order to develop a state of generalized intelligence. One primary difference is that machines function within the parameters of set logics defined by their programming, while humans are able to function in the commonsense world without rational logic—without needing or utilizing a set theory of mind.[3]

Ethics, the study of moral principles, is a system of thought so fully developed and structured as to be rendered almost opaque to those outside the field. In business, as well as in scientific study, ethics is the most commonly applied philosophy used to determine right and wrong. Administration and human resource departments utilize philosophies of ethics to define and contrast moral versus immoral behavior. The only exposure to ethics for most scientists and physicians is most often limited to a listing of rules relating to appropriate and inappropriate behavior. At the limits of science, and at the limits of current research, ethical considerations are far less clear, and far less defined. Technical work, based on sometimes questionable ethics, is progressing at an exponential rate. Examples include the deciphering and use of the genetic code, and the development of artificial CNS zombie systems. In these cases, as in many others, technology is proceeding far faster than our understanding of the biologic and philosophic systems that are being replaced. There is a wide spectrum of multivalent moral questions related to the potential for use and abuse of intelligent machine systems by humans. Socioeconomically, human roles are being replaced with AI algorithms and robotics. AI systems are becoming so increasing complex, it is possible that in the future some may become candidates for having moral status. If superintelligent systems evolve with the capacity to control existence (their own as well as ours), moral complexity increases, and questions of ethics shift from us into the potential behavior of the machines.[4]

Ethical arguments can be made that some AI technologies should not be developed, and that others, particularly the forms that we create, should be monitored closely. But humans are able to function outside logic.

In the near future we are more likely than not to create any system that can be built with the available technology. This is true for areas of focus outside our understanding—even for areas of obvious moral illegitimacy. Artificial CNS constructs (zombie systems) are almost certain to exist in our future.

This final section is an attempt to tie together the science and logic of the previous chapters into an overall gestalt. Chapter 11, Anthropomorphism: Philosophies of AI Dreaming and Consciousness, delves further into the philosophy of AI consciousness—the anthropomorphism of our human experience as related to our interactions with our machines. Chapter 12, Searching for Dreams in Other (Stranger) Places, addresses the methodology used to explore the evidence for dreams outside the biologic arena, applying this approach to the study of petroglyphs. Chapter 13, Machine Consciousness, summarizes our current understanding of machine correlates of consciousness. Chapter 14, Forms of Machine Dreaming, answers the questions at the crux of this book, as to whether machines might actually dream, and how machine dreaming might function. Chapter 15, The Antropomorphic Dream Machine, looks to the future, and what this capacity for dreaming might mean for both machines and humans.

My work and training (Pagel) is as a research scientist and clinician. Philosophy has been an acquired taste, a perspective required in order to understand and somehow order an overview of the science, theories, and research methodologies involved in my chosen fields of study. My training in neurochemistry, electrophysiology, and medicine of sleep came with little exposure to the systemic rigor of philosophic systems of thought. My background in philosophy is therefore self-obtained through reading, discussion, and peer-reviewed publication. Some philosophic systems of understanding seem self-evident. Others, such as ethics, can be particularly difficult to cogently comprehend.

## Notes

1. McCulloch, W., & Pitts, W. (1965). A logical calculus of the ideas immanent in nervous activity. In W. S. McCulloch (Ed.), *Embodiments of mind* (pp. 19−39). Cambridge, MA: MIT Press.
2. Boden, M. (Ed.). (2005). *The philosophy of artificial intelligence* (p. 2). Oxford: Oxford University Press.
3. Dreyfus, H., & Dreyfus, S. (1988). Making a mind versus modeling the brain: Artificial intelligence back at a break point. *Artificial Intelligence, 117*(1), 15−43.
4. Bostrom, N., & Yudkowsky, E. (2014). The ethics of artificial intelligence. In K. Frankish & W. Ramsey (Eds.), *The Cambridge handbook of artificial intelligence* (pp. 316−334). Cambridge: Cambridge University Press.

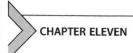

# CHAPTER ELEVEN

# Anthropomorphism: Philosophies of AI Dreaming and Consciousness

*By the poem, "Es et non," which is the "yes" and the "no" of Pythagoras, he understood truth and error in our human knowledge and the profane sciences. Finding that he succeeded in fitting in all these things well to his satisfaction, he was so bold as to feel it was assured that it was the spirit of Truth that by his dream had deigned to open before him the treasures of all the sciences.*

**Rene Descartes (1691).[1]**

Philosophy is a rational and critical human study of basic human principles and concepts. Artificial intelligence (AI) is in its essence a philosophical concept. Using this book as an example, there is not a chapter that does not at some level digress into some form of rational philosophical enquiry. Programming requires the ability to construct logical philosophic formulations that can be consistently interpreted and analyzed by a non-human system. The Turing Test, developed early on in the field, is less a test of whether consciousness has developed within an artificial system, than it is a formed philosophical dynamic that questions the definition of consciousness. Consciousness, even when addressed on a purely operative or mechanistic level, is primarily a philosophic concept. Its definition, its criteria, and its testing are in the philosophic domain, wide open, even after centuries of study, to the critical enquiry and reconsideration of its basic nature, applicable principles, and its aspects.

Consciousness is a basic principle of being. As such, it is a suitable topic for philosophic enquiry and empiric focus. Computer programming and AI are practical and applied offshoots, difficult to discuss without resorting to the use of philosophical knowledge and approaches. Dreams are somewhat different, better viewed as aspects of absolute and relative metaphor. The philosophic discussion of

*Machine Dreaming and Consciousness.*
DOI: http://dx.doi.org/10.1016/B978-0-12-803720-1.00011-6
153

dreaming is most often presented as a construct for untruth, an approach utilized by both Plato and Descartes. More recent philosophers, such as Heidegger, have found further inspiration for the analysis of "truth" in the parable of Plato's Cave, a philosophic construct built upon metaphors of dreaming.[2] It is a paradox that Descartes' initial inspiration for developing the scientific method came from a series of dreams (see initial chapter quote). Today's philosophers, in addressing dreams, tend to address dreams within systems of philosophic doctrine as developed by earlier philosophers, particularly Plato and Descartes. Karl Popper, in his version of scientific philosophy, uses the concept of "falsification," a reconstitution of Descartes vision of the dream as untruth.[3] But in the last 50 years, since REM sleep was discovered, philosophers have presumed the dream state to be a biologic construct, better addressed by neuroscientists than philosophers.[4] Most of today's philosophers incorporate a belief in dream's theoretic neurobiological construct (REMS) into their philosophic approaches to dream.[5]

Dreams are humanly ubiquitous, unique, and personal. And as such, each individual has their own intensely personal concept of dream and the process that is thought of as dreaming. An understanding of dreaming may be based on personal experience, social mores, belief systems, presumed knowledge, literature, and/or shared anecdote. That understanding is rarely based on philosophic enquiry or science. Even when based on "science," the science is often casual, incorrect, or clouded. Neither dream science nor dream philosophy are typically approached with disciplined empirical analysis.[6] While it can be considered quite rational to discuss the possibility of consciousness in a machine (just check the literature index on Google), any discussion of "machine dreaming" is most likely to be presented in the context of fantasy, science fiction, song, economics, or as a computer game, rather than as science.[7]

## ANTHROPOMORPHISM

In any discussion of machine dreaming, the question of anthropomorphism will arise. Anthropomorphism is the cognitive approach that we use in applying our human understandings and schemas as a basis for inferring the properties of nonhuman entities. Such inferences are often far from accurate.[8] Yet it is a human characteristic to anthropomorphize.

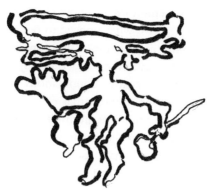

**Figure 11.1** Migrane Man-Mesa Pietra, Trail 6.

Among our oldest artifacts and art (35,000 BC) are anthropomorphic paintings and carved figures, part human and part animal. A significant percentage of petroglyphs are anthropomorphic (Fig. 11.1). Historically, much of our visual art has been anthropomorphic, consisting of portraits, human images, and fantastic human-like images. In today's world, we humans continue to anthropomorphize much of life experience. Beyond anthropomorphizing our pets, we anthropomorphize much of our lives, our knowledge and our beliefs. We approach our waking lives with an anthropomorphic cognitive bias. We are most likely to show this bias in situations in which our knowledge is low and our abilities to have an effect on others is high.[8] We tend to anthropomorphize such situations because each of us has a highly developed social knowledge based on a prolonged schooling in personal human-to-human interactions. From early in life, we are taught to mimic, understand, and communicate with other humans. We know more about other humans than about any other subject. In difficult, poorly described, and poorly understood situations, we extend the depth of our knowledge about humans into our description of nonhuman entities and systems, topics that we understand far less.[9] In interacting with animals, most humans will anthropomorphize, particularly in interacting with their pets. Such a perspective is less common, and often less positive when applied to wild animals. But we typically extend this approach well beyond our interactions with other biological creatures. We create anthropomorphic dolls and stuffed animals that we love and endow with human emotions. We anthropomorphize aspects of our external environment such as the beauty, power, and the malevolence of mountains, oceans, clouds, and sunsets. Anthropomorphic emotions are both positive and negative.

Applied anthropomorphic emotions are most likely to be positive for our pets and toys, and most negative when applied to our machines.[10]

In the scientific community, the use of anthropomorphic language has traditionally been viewed as indicating a lack of objectivity. Scientifically, anthropomorphism has very negative connotations. The term is used in debates and discussion as a direct insult that can be applied to presented data. More directly it can be applied as an insult of the researcher or theorist. Scientists may be warned in their training to avoid assumptions that animals share any of the same mental, social, and emotional capacities of humans.[11] In addressing nonbiologic systems, anthropomorphism is even less well tolerated. Yet despite admonitions, personal and emotional interactions with our machines are quite common.[10]

An example of machine anthropomorphism is the expression or belief that your PC or your cell phone is dysfunctional, in part, because it is angry at you. Another is the suggestion that an intelligent robot would find a human woman sexy and would be driven to mate with her. Predictions about an AI's behavior being either logical, or illogical, can be projections of anthropomorphism.[12] The conscious use of anthropomorphic metaphor can sometimes be appropriate and even useful. Ascribing mental processes to the computer, under the proper circumstances, may serve to help us to understand what the computer will do. How our actions will affect the computer, how to compare computers with ourselves, and conceivably how to design human–compatible computer programs illustrate that, "the trick is to know enough about how humans and computers think to say *exactly* what they have in common, and, when we lack this knowledge, to use the comparison to *suggest* theories of human thinking or computer thinking."[13]

## ANTHROPOMORPHIC FEARS

The human tendency is to ascribe negative aspects and emotions to machines. While there is little question that cognitive extenders such as the personal computer, the Internet, and the cell phone have had positive effects on our behaviors, we are reticent in giving them praise. We attribute negative possibilities—even nightmare scenarios—to conscious machine systems. Self-aware, self-improving AI systems bent on efficiency, self-preservation, and resource acquisition are likely future possibilities. Such systems could be superintelligent and smarter than humans.[14] Our fears lead us to question whether such systems will need or tolerate humans. Will such "nightmare" systems, the offspring of the autonomous drone weapon systems that we have already designed, treat us better than we treat ourselves?

Taken to its extreme, anthropomorphism can become "anthropocentrism." For the anthropocentrist, the external and internal environment is described and defined based purely on the ways in which it can affect humans. Anthropocentrism can be part of belief systems and religious views. It can include the perspective that gods are created in our own human image. From the anthropocentrist perspective, a human should do everything possible to protect and preserve its species. Anthropcentrist behaviors include the destruction of other species (e.g., predator removal) and environmental destruction (e.g., unmitigated resource extraction). An anthropocentrist might reject claims that the Earth's resources are limited or that unchecked human population growth will exceed the carrying capacity of Earth and result in wars and famines as resources become scarce.[15] Anthropocentrism can be used to support the concept that human-based collateral damage is justified even its most extreme forms (e.g., planetary destruction secondary to human warfare or environmental manipulation).

## ANTHROPOMORPHIC MACHINES

The field of robotics has invested heavily in anthropomorphic body patterns, even when they are not functionally required. In human–robotic interactions, studies seem to indicate that cooperation and learning can be facilitated when the robot has an anthropomorphic appearance.[16] In user interactions, humans can sometimes, however, exhibit negative social and emotional responses as well as decreased trust towards robots that closely, but imperfectly, resemble humans. Negative reactions are most likely to occur when human users encounter proactive behavior on the part of a robot that does not respect a safety distance. In situations in which a robot is present but has no particular use, negative feelings are also more likely to be expressed.[17]

Our fears of machine systems may in part be due to a lack of emotional feedback. The behavioral expression of emotion is within the capacity of robotic systems. Happy images and smolgies as part of the interface add the possibility for positive anthropomorphic interactions parodying the same interactions we had as children with our dolls and teddy bears. Systems utilizing positive emotional cues in toys such as "Tickle me Elmo" have been incredibly popular. It is fairly easy to have anger towards a disembodied Internet or a plastic computer. We seem to be able to maintain better attitudes towards those more entrancingly designed. Apple Corporation emphasizes this design approach. It is not nearly so easy to have anger towards an object designed to enhance affection. Anthropomorphic metaphors, used inappropriately, can lead us to develop false beliefs about the behavior of computers.

## ANTROPOMORPHISM AS A MARKER FOR CONSCIOUSNESS

The ability to develop and use the anthropomorphic perspective has been proposed as a maker for semantic consciousness. Heinz Pagels refers to any system that expresses anthropomorphism as an "intentional engine," a system that has beliefs, emotions, exercises free will, and the capacity for representing meaning.[10] If the ability to assume the human-based anthropomorphic role is the key marker for human-equivalent consciousness, there is less chance that a nonbiologic machine system might develop consciousness.[18] Any system that cannot assume an anthropomorphic perspective might also be unable to adequately appreciate us, their creators. Such a lack of appreciation for all things human could potentially produce a situation in which a created machine system had no interest in maintaining human domination. It has been suggested that such a machine-based insight could precipitate the end of the human era.[14] Our fears lead us to require anthropomorphism in our creations. Among the first to address this issue was not a philosopher, but rather the writer of science fiction, Issac Asimov, who in 1941 famously postulated the three required laws of robotics:

1. A robot may not injure a human being or, through inaction, allow a human being to come to harm;
2. A robot must obey any orders given to it by human beings, except where such orders would conflict with the First Law; and
3. A robot must protect its own existence as long as such protection does not conflict with the First or Second Laws (Asimov-I Robot).[19]

Asimov's laws of robotics are anthropocentric. They incorporate our fears of creating a machine that is more intelligent, more physically beautiful, and more functional. These laws are based on our perceived need for protection from such systems. Anthropocentrism is an attempt to place and maintain the human at the center of the robot's universe, preserving our role as the one responsible for setting goals, determining outcomes, and judging consequences. From the anthropocentric perspective, it is only with such tightly programmed control that we might be assured of safety and comfort in interacting with anthropomorphically conscious machines.

## ANTHROPOMORPHIC DREAMS

If dreaming is something that only a human can do, the postulate that a machine might dream becomes an impossibility. This definition for dreaming makes it logically impossible that either a machine or a nonhuman animal would be able to dream. As applied to our machines, this assertion of anthropocentrism reflects a thinly veiled fear of a future in which we, as a species, might no longer be preeminent. What if machines are dreaming? There is good evidence that some humans never recall dreams (i.e., there is no evidence to indicate that they are actually dreaming).[20] The scientific interest in dreaming that peaked during the Freudian and REM sleep eras is in decline.[21] And for many in today's modern world, dreams are often viewed as psuedoscience. Or totally ignored. It is as if we are intentionally delegating the capacity to dream to our creations, while losing our own interest in and capacity to dream.

For Descartes the dreamer, yes could be no, and truth derivative from error. Waking truth was evident because it lacked the irrationality and inconsistency of dream. What is supersedes what is not ("non" is clearly secondary to "es"). This is the anthropomorphic world in which we live. No longer needing dreams, what then becomes of our specialness, our ability to see so many sides of each issue, and our ability to constantly change and develop. Even for the true anthropocentrist, the loss of such an irrational process as dreaming might actually matter. Without the ability to use and actualize our dreams, we will lose capacity for emotional processing and insight into our behaviors. We will lose aspects of our creativity. We will be losing an aspect that is essential to our humanity.

# Notes

1. Descartes, R. (1691). Descartes three-fold dream. In *La vie de Monsieur Des-Cartes* (A. Baillet, Trans., pp. 81–86). Paris: Chez Daniel Horthemels.
2. Plato (380 BC) The cave: The first stage. *The Republic.* Rouse, W. H. D. (Ed.). (2008). *The Republic: Book VII* (pp. 365–401). New York: Penguin Group Inc.

   *Picture people dwelling in an underground chamber like a cave, with a long entrance open to the light on its entire width. In this chamber people are shackled at their legs and necks from childhood, so that they remain in the same spot, and look only at what is in front of them, at what is present before them. Because of their shackles they are unable to turn their heads. However, light reaches them from behind, from a fire burning up higher and at a distance. Between the fire and the prisoners, behind their backs, runs a path along which a small wall has been built, like the screen at a puppet shows between the exhibitors and their audience, and above which they, the puppeteers, show their artistry. I see, he says. Imagine further that there are people carrying all sorts of things along behind the screen, projecting above it, including figures of men and animals made of stone and wood, and all sorts of other man-made artifacts. Naturally, some of these people would be talking among themselves, and others would be silent.*

   *A peculiar picture you have drawn, and peculiar prisoners!*

   *They are very much like us! Now tell me, do you think such people could see anything, whether on their own account or with the help of their fellows, except the shadows thrown by the fire on the wall of the cave opposite them?*

   Passage addressed in detail as associated with dreaming and the search for truth: Heidegger, M. (2002). *The essence of truth.* London: Continuum; Pagel, J. F. (2008). *The limits of dream: A scientific exploration of the mind/brain interface.* Oxford: Academic Press.
3. Popper, K. (1934). Falsification versus conventionalism. In D. Miller (Ed.), *Popper selections* (pp. 143–151). Princeton, NJ: Princeton University Press.
4. Pagel, J. F. (2008). *The limits of dream: A scientific exploration of the mind/brain interface.* Oxford: Academic Press.
5. Chambers, D. (1996). *The conscious mind: In search of a fundamental theory.* New York: Oxford University Press.
6. Foulks, D. (1993). Functions of dreaming. In A. Moffit, M. Kramer, & R. Hoffmann (Eds.), *The functions of dreaming* (pp. 11–20). Albany, NY: SUNY Press.
7. Phillips, J., & Mertz, J. (1984). *Machine dreams* (novel); Mirowski, P. (2002). *Machine dreams: Economics becomes cyborg science* (non-fiction); Little Dragon (2009). *Machine dreams* (studio album) Peace Frog; Hashio Shoho Neko (2015). *Machine dreams* (hover video game).
8. Hutson, M. (2012). *The 7 laws of magical thinking: How irrational beliefs keep us happy, healthy, and sane* (pp. 165–181). New York: Hudson Street Press.
9. Epley, N., Waytz, A., & Cacioppo, J. T. (2007). On seeing human: A three-factor theory of anthropomorphism. *Psychological Review, 114*(4), 864–886.
10. Pagels, H. (1988). *The dreams of reason: The computer and the rise of the sciences of complexity* (p. 230). New York: Bantam Books.
11. Flynn, C. (2008). *Social creatures: A human and animal studies reader.* New York: Lantern Books.
12. Yudkowsky, E. (2008). Artificial intelligence as a positive and negative factor in global risk. In N. Bostrom & M. Cirkovic (Eds.), *Global catastrophic risks.* Oxford: Oxford University Press.

13. Cohen, P., & Feigenbaum, E. (Eds.). (2014). *The handbook of artificial intelligence* (Vol. 3). Oxford: Butterworth-Heinemann.
14. Barrat, J. (2013). *Our final invention: Artificial intelligence and the end of the human era.* New York: Tomas Dunne Books.
15. Boddice, R. (Ed.). (2011). *Anthropocentrism: Humans, animals, environments.* Leiden and Boston, MA: Brill.
16. Zlotowski, J., Proudfoot, D., Yogeeswaran, K., & Bartneck, C. (2015). Anthropomorphism: Opportunities and challenges in human—robot interaction. *International Journal of Social Robotics, 7*(3), 347—360.
17. Mathur, M. B., & Reichling, D. B. (2016). Navigating a social world with robot partners: A quantitative cartography of the uncanny valley. *Cognition, 146,* 22—32.
18. Demasio, A. (1999). *The feeling of what happens: Body and emotion in the making of consciousness.* San Diego, CA: Harcourt Inc.
19. Asimov, I. (1941/1950). *I robot.* New York: Gnome Press.
20. Pagel, J. F. (2003). Non-dreamers. *Sleep Medicine, 4,* 235—241.
21. Pagel, J. F. (2010). Preface. In *Dreaming and nightmares. Sleep Medicine Clinics, 5*(2). Philadelphia, PA: Saunders/Elsevier.

# CHAPTER TWELVE

# Searching for Dreams in Other (Stranger) Places

*I met a traveller from an antique land*
*Who said: Two vast and trunkless legs of stone*
*Stand in the desert. Near them on the sand,*
*Half sunk, a shatter'd visage lies, whose frown*
*And wrinkled lip and sneer of cold command*
*Tell that its sculptor well those passions read*
*Which yet survive, stamp'd on these lifeless things,*
*The hand that mock'd them and the heart that fed.*
*And on the pedestal those words appear:*
*"My name is Ozymandis, king of kings:*
*Look on my works, ye mighty, and despair!"*
*Nothing beside remains: round the decay*
*Of that colossal wreck, boundless and bare,*
*The lone and level sands stretch far away.*

*Percy Shelley-Ozymandis.*[1]

Dreams exist outside the biology of an organism. Dream-based images are part of the spectrum of renderings that we call art. In the last hundred years, the attempt to create artificial dreams has become part of our technology, in photographs, in film, and now in AI. Artists and technicians sometimes comment on how they used dreams in their process of creation, or explain how and why they chose to integrate dream-like effects in their creative work. But there are many dream-like that remain unlabeled as to their origin. Working back from what we know about humans and their utilization of dream imagery, we can make reasonable assumptions as to which might have been inspired by dreams. Carl Jung was one of the first clinician-scientists attempting to make such analysis, searching for dream-inspired symbols in recorded history and art.[2] A similar methodology can be used to search for dream-based patterns—outside biology, and outside human reports—in symbols and images that date back to the Paleolithic era and our species' first transition to reflexive consciousness.

*Machine Dreaming and Consciousness.*
DOI: http://dx.doi.org/10.1016/B978-0-12-803720-1.00012-8

## THE CAVE ART OF SOUTHWEST EUROPE

There are very few decorated human artifacts that predate the paintings of Chauvet Cave in Southern France (created 32,000 years ago).[3] In caves from this region our *Homo sapiens* ancestors drew mystical creatures: pregnant mares, now extinct ibexes, dancing cave bears, mastodons, and charging rhinoceroses, as well as occasional anthropomorphic images of humans. From this Paleolithic era, archeologists have discovered the first elaborate burials and the first evidence of refined, decorated, and nonutilitarian tools. So far as we know, none of the other protohumans, including the Neanderthals, created images other than handprints.[4] The attribute of creating art and decoration is among the primary characteristics that can be used to archeologically differentiate our species.[5]

Anthropologist Claude Levi-Strauss points out that our only access to the Paleolithic mind is through the close examination and analysis of the products of those minds.[6] In the analysis of the cave paintings, we see indications that these protohumans were likely to have been self-aware, with the capacity to view themselves as independent of one another and the world around them. The paintings indicate that the painters conceived of themselves as different from other animals Fig. 1.1. Further analysis suggests that the cave-painters had the capacity for reflexive consciousness—the ability to recognize that the thinking subject had his or her own acts, existing within a socially based self-hood affecting others. Such an awareness may be what differentiated our ancestors from the other protomodern humans.[7] We might recognize these Paleolithic hunters, even today, as human.[8] The cave paintings are the best evidence we have that our ancestors developed convergent and divergent forms of reflexive consciousness—core processes of modern creativity.[9]

The use of dreams is a widely recognized and valued part of artistic rendering in virtually every cultural community populating this planet.[10] Jung's work suggests that dream incorporation into art may be a basic human characteristic.[2] The power that the cave paintings exert on the viewer today can be no less than the power they had to affect the Paleolithic viewer who carried flickering lights deep into the absolute darkness, to confront imagined images from beyond their waking reality.[11]

Part of being human has been to be fascinated by dreams. Dreaming is an inspiration for individual- and species-based creativity. Our dreams provide us with the ability to find alterative approaches to functioning in the external world. It is very likely that it was our dreams that provided the inspiration, the ecstasy, and the possibility for such remarkable creations as the cave paintings.[12] It is quite possible that reflexive consciousness and the capability to create such art would not be possible if our ancestors had not developed the capacity to dream.[3,11] Arguments supporting the potential role for dreams in Paleolithic cave art are summarized in Table 12.1.

## DREAMS IN ART

It is very likely that some of the Paleolithic cave art images were inspired by dreams. Carl Jung, in his surveys of Eastern and Western art, searched art for the culturally shared symbols that he called archetypes. He had learned from his mentor, Sigmund Freud, to search for sexual symbols in art—church steeples, elongated forms, caverns, and holes. But Jung extended his index of dream symbols beyond the sexual. Based on the Eastern art of the mandala, he proposed that circle forms were often unconscious depictions of the soul.[2] For Jung, the psychoanalyst and theorist, much of creative art was unconscious, and in being unconscious, was likely derived from dream.[13] In the 19th century, artists such as Goya and

**Table 12.1** Summary of evidence that dreams contributed to Paleolithic cave paintings

— Dreams are a virtually ubiquitous human experience.
— Cave site design likely reflects the Paleolithic understanding of the nether world—darkness requiring artificial lighting with paintings that appear to move in this light, entrance chambers and deeper passages leading to panels of the art that incorporate the rocks and protrusions of the caves into its motif.
— The paintings are representational rather than perceptual—high-quality non-naturalistic, and multidimensional, incorporating multiperspectives, apparent motion, and storylines; artistic qualities that suggest incorporation of altered states of consciousness in their creation.
— Visually, dream imagery utilizes a cognitive paradigm that includes the transformation of representational images from three- to two-dimensional status incorporating aspects of point of view, perspective, and placement of imagery.
— At their furthest and darkest reaches, the paintings include bizarre images of themes including human–animal transformations, death, and sexuality—emotional and significant content typical of dreams and nightmares.
— Historically persistent hunting-gathering cultures often have a dream-associated shamanistic focus that may include ritual and practice involving cave art and paintings.
— An identifiable primary function of dreaming is in the creative process, and even today most artists utilize dream input in their work.

Ruselli painted works derived from their dreams. Since that time, surrealism, Da Da, expressionism, and impressionism have celebrated dream-like qualities and incorporated dream experiences. Photographers and filmmakers adapted developing technologies into the creation of dream-like visuals. Today, many successful artists incorporate dream imagery into their work. Dream-associated phenomena are present in almost all forms of art.[9] It is rare to find a visual artist who does not at least occasionally use their dreams.[14] Juried shows and Internet competitions address works derived from dream.[15] And, there are many artists, particularly those who have experienced major physical and/or emotional trauma, who use the distressing dreams of nightmare to produce their most powerful works.[16] In today's artistic world, just as in the Paleolithic, dreams and nightmares are used creatively in the inspiration and enhancement of artistic works.

## PETROGLYPHS

Near the modern Pueblo of Okay Owinge, in Northern New Mexico, is Mesa Pietra—a site with one of the longest histories of continuous human occupation for any area in North America. There, more than 80,000 engravings and images have been picked into the dark basalt boulders of an ancient lava flow. Recent images include tagging, graffiti, and traced initials (Fig. 12.1). Others are historic, dating from the era of the early railroad, sheepherders, and from workers at the local WPA

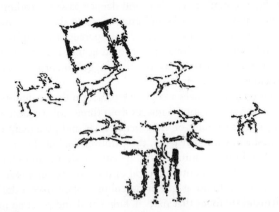

**Figure 12.1** Graffiti on Pueblo era petroglyphs. Big Arsenic site—Rio Grade del Norte National Monument.

camp. Slightly older images date from first Western contact, including portraits of Spanish soldiers, priests, directionally set compasses, figures wearing clothes, Christian crosses, and horses. The majority of images ($\sim 80\%$) were produced during the Pueblo era (AD 1300−1600) when at least a dozen large pueblos surrounded the site.[17] Unlike Shelly's Ozymandus, these images are not labeled with a pronouncement as to their significance. As we currently understand many of these images are ritualistic, marking the limits of native hunting and living range.[18] The images include depictions of birth, death, puberty, triumph, failure, and religious ecstasy. Some images are spirals marking astronomical time.

This site also includes other, far more ancient images, dating back to the Archaic era (6,000−10,000 years ago). The Archaic era is marked in time by spear points, sometimes found as part of Ice Age Mastodon kills. Images, inscribed on ancient shrine sites such as Lightening Rock, are far different from more modern renderings. Except for the occasional hand-prints, these petroglyphs are primarily wandering lines and grids. Again, what remains is all that we can use in our attempts to understand the minds of their creators.[6] The creators of these images considered and described their world in a different fashion than we typically do today.[9]

## SEARCHING FOR DREAM IMAGES

Today dreams are often an inspiration for visual art. Since some of the cave paintings of Southwest Europe are likely to have been based on dreams. It is quite likely that some of the more than 80,000 images at Mesa Pietra are dream-based. There are typical patterns of phenomenology asso-ciated with artistic works that are known to have been derived from dream. This perspective can be applied to petroglyphs in the attempt to discover which images are most likely to have been derived from dream.

It is a primary characteristic of dream content that it has continuity with waking experience. Any images derived from dream should reflect their creators' waking life. Pueblo era depictions from daily life, including hunting, fighting, or playing music, are more likely to be dream-based than are unusual geometric forms. These anthropomorphic images that involve waking activities are often interpreted by archeologists as provid-ing some degree of insight into daily life.[19] Some of these images may have come from dreams.

Another primary dream characteristic is that of being an individual rather than a shared experience. Since dream-based images are individual rather than collective, they are often unique. Uniqueness as a dream characteristic is similar to bizarreness, a dream characteristic that has been extensively studied. Dream bizarreness is characterized by discontinuity, incongruity, and uncertainty (Hobson), and/or confusion and bizarre personification (Hunt).[20] In a search for petroglyphs that are potentially dream-based, uniqueness is a primary criteria. At Mesa Pietra, most images are repeated: animals, tracks, hand- and footprints, flute players, Venus stars, shields, vulva representations, spirals, and crosses (Fig. 12.1). Because they are not unique, it is doubtful that these typical and repeated patterns would be derived from dreams. While there are repetitive anthropomorphic images (e.g., man with shield, woman giving birth), human forms are the images that are most likely to be unique, each different from the other. Like dreams, these images were created by humans. They are anthropomorphic images from the Anthropocene—the age of humans. Dreams are anthropocentric, in that the dreamer is almost always present in the dream, sometimes only as a point of view, but at other times in full lucid control of the dream experience. It would not be surprising that a dream-based petroglyph would include an image of the dreamer (Fig. 10.1 and 11.1).

Dreams include complex, emotional, and changing images integrated with metaphorical and associative memories. This content is developed on awakening into a narrative story. Petroglyph images are most often static. The cave paintings include depth of field, point of view, and multiple lining, all techniques that can be used to portray a sense of both movement and story—all techniques difficult to incorporate into a petroglyph.[21] But even pecked, static images can tell stories. There are women giving birth, there is dancing and music being played, men waving shields, and upside-down men falling from rock faces.

There are powerful images, conveying both motion and story, from the period of first contact. Historically the Mesa Pietra Site was part of the Pueblo Revolt, when in the Late 1600s the native tribes rebelled, attacked, and evicted the Spanish. The Spanish returned in a bloody reconquest. As historically recorded at the Acoma Pueblo, soldiers cut the right foot from every male of potential fighting age. Horrified and intimidated, the Pueblos once again came under Spanish rule.[22] Oral histories suggest that the Pueblo at Mesa Pietra was subjected to the same mutilations. There are several petroglyphic panels that appear to be markers for

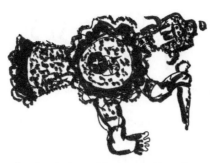

**Figure 12.2** One-legged crying turkey with dagger. Mesa Pietra.

this event: a one-legged man with a cross on his shoulder (Fig. 10.1); an image of what appears to be the Spanish Lion being strangled by a snake; and most powerful, being a one-legged turkey holding a dagger over its head. A large tear drips down its face (Fig. 12.2). This image meets other dream-based criteria. Dream content is most often emotionally negative (>60%), a characteristic particularly true for images produced by individuals that have experienced major trauma. Such nightmares often include aspects of the actual experience of trauma presented within a powerful contextual image.[23]

The meaning of a dream-based image is rarely obvious. It requires interpretation. Many of the anthropomorphic petroglyph images are sexually explicit, fitting into psychoanalytic perspectives (>70% are impossibly well-endowed males, and many repeated vulva images). There are circle shields and spirals, and, most intriguingly, there are the depictions of circles (babies) being born. This, of course, begs the question as to who first came to interpret the circle as an image representing the soul. Jung stayed for a time just across the river at the Los Luceros Hacienda shortly before he developed and published his theories of archetypes.[24]

The meaning, function, and basis of petroglyph imagery remains a matter of contention. This is particularly true for the early Archaic Mesa Pietra images. The early images—wandering lines, grids, and patterns—could be maps or patterns observed in the stars. They might be meditative reflections of retinal blood vessels, or eye floaters.[12] They could reflect the structure and form underlying imagery, such as seen in abstract expressionist paintings (e.g., the grids of Agnes Martin). These ancient markings are what our ancient ancestors inscribed on these rocks for us to see. Like dreams, these grids and lines could mark the perceived

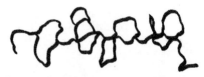

**Figure 12.3** An Archaic era petroglyph. Mesa Pietra, Trail 6.

portal into another form of consciousness. It is not their creators' problem that we are unable to comprehend (Fig. 12.3).

Each petroglyph forms data pecked in digital code, the 0 removed, the 1 left in place. Viewed as such, each petroglyph includes bits of this digital/pixel code. A subset of images, particularly those from early contact, have a phenomenology characteristic of dream-based art. As based on this site's history, it is difficult to conceive of the image of the crying, one-legged turkey as being anything other than a nightmare image produced after the experience of trauma. This image has multiple attributes that are typical of dream images:

1. It has continuity with life experience;
2. It is unique and individual—there are no other petroglyphs depicting crying, one-legged turkeys;
3. It tells an emotional, complex, and continuing story. The tear will always be falling. Just across the highway from the site a guard posted by the Conquistador's Statue attempts to keep away locals determined cut off its right foot;
4. It is a dark and negative depiction of experienced trauma and nightmare;
5. It is anthropomorphic, with its dismembered sacrificial turkey holding a dagger in his hand.

While there is no caption at the base of the petroglyph, no verbal or written human report, the evidence strongly suggests that this petroglyph is likely to have been inspired by a nightmare.

## OTHER PLACES FOR DREAM PHENOMENOLOGY— MACHINES

This methodological approach can be used to search for evidence of dreaming outside the human biologic construct. Archeologists confronted with such a statue as Shelley's Ozymandis, standing in the desert untitled and unexplained, would likely decide to limit their assessment to the physical evidence of the time and method of creation, and perhaps to any associated and concrete artifacts. But even so, Ozymandis—King of

**Table 12.2** Dream-associated phenomenology association with Paleolithic cave paintings and prehistoric North American rock art (petroglyphs)

| Cave paintings | Petroglyphs | Machine dream equivalents |
|---|---|---|
| Anthopomorphism | Anthropomorphism | ★★ |
| Uniqueness (bizarreness) | Uniqueness (bizarreness) | ★★ |
| Representational imagery | Representational imagery | ★★ |
| Interpretation required | Interpretation required | ★★ |
| Creative aesthetic | Creative aesthetic | + / − |
| Ecstatic component to art | Less ecstatic component | − |
| Metaphoric stories | Metaphoric stories | − |
| Negative content | Negative content | − |
| Trauma association (specific works) | Trauma association (specific works) | − |
| Sleep correlate (sited in darkness) | − | − |
| Shamanistic focus | Shamanistic focus | − |

Areas and the degree of possible machine correlation are noted (−, + / −, ★, ★★).

Kings—would still be surveying his dreams of creation and despair, mocking them with his hand, and his passions, the heart that fed them.

One way to approach the possibility that dreaming was involved in the creation of prehistoric artistic renderings is to assess for the presence and/or absence of suggested dream correlates (Table 12.2).

Machine dream equivalents share phenomenologic characteristics with art derived from the biologic experience of dreaming. The machine dream equivalents discussed in this book are often anthropomorphic, addressing human issues and utilizing human databases. The data results produced by neural net systems and nonparametic, fuzzy logic programming can be unique, hallucinatory, possibly creative, and apparently non-applicable to the set-goal of analysis—much like the dreams incorporated into and inspiring art. The visual imagery derived from dream is most often representational (nonperceptually based), as are dream-based petroglyphs and machine-constructed images. Like dreams, petroglyphs and complexly portrayed machine images are difficult to understand and often require interpretation. These characteristics are shared by dream reports, purportedly dream-based petroglyph images, and machine dream-equivalent states.

But some of the characteristics shared between dreams and the petroglyphs that seem most clearly dream-based, such as the one-legged turkey, are not evident for machines. Machine dream equivalents such as the

GOOGLE dreams and climate data are rarely aesthetically beautiful.[25] There is little about computer-developed images that suggests an ecstatic component. And while apparent emotional expression can be technically created, there is nothing to suggest that such expressions are somehow reflective of underlying emotional psychodynamics equivalent to the human dream and nightmare process.

Paleolithic, Archaic, and prehistoric rock-art is likely to incorporate inspiration and experience derived from dreams. Some of the same dream-associated characteristics are also present in machine dream equivalents. Dream-inspired paintings and petroglyphs, however, demonstrate dream phenomena that are not present in machines. Dream-based art incorporates ecstasy, creative aesthetic, metaphors formed into stories, and evidence for psychodynamic emotional processing. These executive-level and tertiary consciousness aspects of dreaming have been difficult to scientifically address and study. Undoubtedly important, these basic characteristics define our humanity. Yet these topics are rarely the focus of scientific inquiry. They are more likely to be addressed in studies of art, the humanities, literature, film, and human psychodynamics. The expression and study of these areas of dream-associated phenomenology is limited, at this point in time, to areas that focus on the expressions of the human mind.

## Notes

1. Shelley, P. (1826). Ozymandias. In *Miscellaneous and posthumous poems of Percy Bysshe Shelley* (p. 100). London: W. Benbow.
2. Jung, C. (1936). Individual dream symbolism in relation to alchemy. In J. Campbell (Ed.), *The portable Jung* (1971 reprint ed., pp. 323–455). New York: Penguin Books.
3. Lewis-Williams, J. (2002). *The mind in the cave: Consciousness and the origins of art.* London and New York: Thames and Hudson.
4. Curtis, G. (2006). *The cave painters: Probing the mysteries of the worlds finest artists.* New York: Anchor Books.
5. de Beaune, S. (2009). Technical invention in the Paleolithic: What if the explanation comes from the cognitive and neuropsychological sciences? In S. de Beaune, F. Coolidge, & T. Wynn (Eds.), *Cognitive archeology and human evolution* (pp. 3–14). Cambridge: Cambridge University Press.
6. Levi-Strauss, C. (1968). *Structural anthropology* (C. Jacobson & B. Grundfest-Schoepf, Trans.). London: Penguin.
7. Finlayson, C. (2009). *The humans who went extinct: Why neanderthals died out and we survived.* Oxford: Oxford University Press.
8. Wynn, T., & Coolidge, F. (2009). Implications for a strict standard for recognizing modern cognition in prehistory. In S. de Beaune, F. Coolidge, & T. Wynn (Eds.), *Cognitive archeology and human evolution* (pp. 117–127). Cambridge: Cambridge University Press.

9. Kyriacou, A. (2009). Innovation and creativity: A neuropsychological perspective. In S. de Beaune, F. Coolidge, & T. Wynn (Eds.), *Cognitive archeology and human evolution* (pp. 15—24). Cambridge: Cambridge University Press; Laming-Emperaire, A. (1959). *Lascaux: Paintings and engravings* (E. Armstrong, Trans.). Baltimore, MD: Penguin Books.

10. Van de Castle, R. (1994). *Our dreaming mind: A sweeping exploration of the role that dreams have played in politics, art, religion, and psychology, from ancient civilizations to the present day.* New York: Ballantine Books; Buckley, K. (2009). *Dreaming and the world's religions.* New York: New York University Press.

11. Gamble, C. (2007). *Origins and revolutions: Human identity in earliest prehistory.* Cambridge: Cambridge University Press.

12. Pagel, J. F. (2014). *Dream science: Exploring the forms of consciousness.* Oxford: Academic Press (Elsevier).

13. Jung, C. (1974). *Dreams* (R. Hull, Trans.). Princeton, NJ: Princeton University Press (Original work published 1961).

14. Pagel, J. F., & Kwiatkowski, C. F. (2003). Creativity and dreaming: Correlation of reported dream incorporation into awake behavior with level and type of creative interest. *Creativity Research Journal, 15*(2&3), 199—205.

15. Pagel, J. F. The Creative Nightmare. (2016) *Dreamtime Magazine.* www.asdreams.org/dreamtime-magazine. Accessed 18.10.16.

16. Pagel, J. F., Kwiatkowski, C., & Broyles, K. (1999). Dream use in film making. *Dreaming, 9*(4), 247—296.

17. Wells, K. (2009). *Life on the rocks: One woman's adventure in petroglyph preservation.* Abequerque, NM: University of New Mexico Press. Mesa Prieta Petroglyph Project—Home, www.mesaprietapetroglyphs.org. Accessed 26.10.16. This site provides information as to how to set up a visit to the site. This book's author (Pagel) is but one of those who guide tours of the site. He also monitors this site as well as the Big Arsenic shrine site in Rio Grande del Norte National Monument for problems of vandalism through Site Watch New Mexico.

18. Palmer, K. (1977). Myth, ritual and rock art. *Archeology and Physical Anthropology in Oceania, 12,* 1—79.

19. Copeland, J. (2008). The rock art of the Dinetah. In *La Pintura: American Rock Art Research Association newsletter* (pp. 7—9, Vol. 34). Tucson, AZ: American Rock Art Research Association.

20. Hobson, J., Hoffman, S., Helfrand, R., & Kostner, D. (1987). Dream bizarreness and the activation synthesis hypothesis. *Human Neurobiology, 6,* 157—164; Hunt, H. (1989). *The multiplicity of dreams.* New Haven, CT: Yale University Press.

21. Whitley, D. (2009). Cave paintings and the human spirit: The origin of creativity and belief. Amherst, NY: Prometheus Books.

22. Wilcox, M. (2009). *The Pueblo Revolt and the Mythology of conquest: An Indigenous Archaeology of Contact.* Berkeley, CA: University of California Press.

23. Hartmann, E. (1998). *Dream and nightmares: The new theory on the origin and meaning of dreams.* New York: Plenum Trade.

24. Deloria, V. (2009). *C.G. Jung and the Sioux traditions: Dreams, visions, nature and the primitive.* New Orleans, LA: Spring Journal Books. Jung also visited Taos Pueblo on his journey to New Mexico where he was invited, as were very few other white men, to visit the circular kivas.

25. Google's AI can dream and here's what it look's like. *IFL Science.* www.iflscience.com/technology/artificial-intelligence-dreams. Accessed 16.10.16.

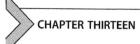

CHAPTER THIRTEEN

# Machine Consciousness

*In fact, the Internet has grown so large and complex that, even though it is constructed from a collection of man-made, largely deterministic parts, we have come to view it almost as a living organism or natural phenomenon that is to be studied.*

*Peterson and Davie (2000).*[1]

Machine consciousness is usually addressed within the construct of autonomous artificial intelligence (AI) systems that have the capacity for self-learning. Today's systems, however, extend well beyond the hardware and controlling software of any circumscribed entity. In these complex systems, hardware, software, memory, and interface comingle into an integrated system in which programmed control is present at all levels. In previous chapters, we have discussed the possibility that dream-like processing can occur in the hardware, in the software programming, in the integrated soft/hardware system of the Internet, and in the sensors and behavioral interaction at the interface. As noted in Chapter 2: The Mechanics of Human Consciousness, consciousness is almost impossible to define generally. Most philosophers and neuroscientists have chosen to approach consciousness from within the limits of established constraints and attributes that can be approached and studied. At various times, from varying perspectives, consciousness has been considered to include intelligence, attention, intention, volition, autonomy, self-awareness, the capacity to self-learn, metacognition, and the ability to rise above programming.

## THE CONSCIOUSNESS OF FINITE STATE MACHINES

Independently operating finite state machines (FSMs) have the capacity to meet some of the criteria set as attributes of human-equivalent consciousness. Consciousness was at one time equated with

*Machine Dreaming and Consciousness.*
DOI: http://dx.doi.org/10.1016/B978-0-12-803720-1.00013-X
175

intelligence. But that argument is presented only rarely today, in part because FSMs have been quite successful in accomplishing the goals set as tests for intelligence. Game-playing systems with access to an applicable database are superior to masters-level human competition in almost all applied tests of intelligence (checkers, backgammon, jeopardy, scrabble, chess, go, etc.).[2] While humans can still occasionally defeat artificial gaming systems, it seems clear that these systems are in the process of surpassing human capacities in the areas of intelligence dependent on memory access and applied intellectual analysis.[3] Language, formal reasoning, planning, mathematics, and game playing require the ability and the intelligence to abstract and process symbols in a logical fashion. Computers are extremely good at such tasks, accomplishing them through the algorithmic manipulation of symbols.[4]

Multifaceted focused attention, as a property of consciousness, can be better accomplished by machines than by most biologic systems including our own. Artificial sensors have supra-human capacity to react and respond to data presented beyond the human sensory range. Such sensor capacity, when combined with an ability to constantly monitor and respond to data, has produced systems that are able to function in all of the areas of attentional focus (executive attention, alerting, and orienting).[5] The machine interface is routinely utilized in attention training for children, brain-damaged individuals, and for individuals with a variety of psychiatric diagnoses in which difficulties in developing and maintaining attentional focus have led to functional limitations.[6]

Intentionality, as an aspect of consciousness, can be artificially parodied.[7] It is a primary characteristic of parametrically programmed FSMs. The process of intention is electronically present in most artificial systems that are able to process information numerically. Humans commonly attribute intentional status to their interactive FSM systems.[8] However, when the definition of intention is anthropomorphically expanded to include the human capacities for belief, intent, or causality, intention (as redefined) becomes impossible for artificial systems.[9]

Some FSM systems, as currently designed, have been able to develop remarkable levels of autonomy within the delineated constraints of their programming. In space, in isolated locales, and when utilized in limited roles in such applications as motor vehicles, appliances, and manufacturing, FSM systems can operate independently of programmer input for extended periods of time. In many areas of medicine, surgical and technological assessment systems require system/body awareness in order to function. Phenomenological self-representation can also be inferred from the ability of some systems to format and develop computer-presented narratives.[10]

Beyond body/system self-awareness, the metacognitive property of "awareness of being aware" has been proposed as a marker that would indicate the capacity of an artificially created system to transcend programming. It is suggested that such metaconsciousness might mark the development of human-like consciousness in machines.[11] There is no clear indication that any currently designed and constructed system has developed an awareness of being aware.

In order to develop the conscious capacity for volition, as a marker for consciousness, an AI system would need to define and readjust its own rules towards its own development. This self-controlled capacity for self-defined learning is sometimes called coherent extrapolated volition (CEV).[12] While attempts are currently being made to endow self-learning AI systems with this capacity, there is little if any evidence that any of these systems have been able to rise above their programming.[13]

Anthropomorphic robot systems are being designed to have the potential capacity to mimic both the physiognomy and behaviors of the human. Such a system might have the capacity to mimic human consciousness and behavior (see HBO's "Westworld"). But at this point in time, such machine capacity must be relegated to the realms of science fiction. The current capacity for FSM systems to attain attributes of consciousness are summarized in Table 13.1.

## SELF-LEARNING AI

As currently designed, self-learning AI systems work to achieve programmed goals. Systems using artificial neural network hardware have demonstrated the capacity to outperform typical digital operating systems when utilized in commonsense human environments. Self-learning systems can be constructed that utilize fuzzy logics, list logics, and looser philosophic logic as software structures. As currently designed, these systems have shown a capacity to respond to changing environmental conditions that is sometimes better than that accomplished by parametrically logical systems.[14]

**Table 13.1** Current FSM capacities in achieving defined aspects of consciousness

| Aspects of consciousness | FSM capacity |
| --- | --- |
| Intelligence | High, in specific areas such as game-playing and data analysis already in excess of normal human capacity |
| Attention | Supra-human based on sensor capacity and capacity for attentional focus |
| Intention | Potentially equivalent to human—as based on programming |
| Self-awareness | Utilized in robotic systems |
| Autonomy | This is a proven capacity for independently operating systems in specific areas of focus |
| Ability to self-learn | Goal defined in some AI systems programmed for such a capacity |
| Metacognition (awareness of being aware) | Not present |
| Volition | Not present |
| Intent/causality | Not present |
| Ability to rise above programming | Not present |
| Ability to mimic human physiognomy and behavior | Limited |

The next level of neural network-based AI will be to extend beyond multilevel networks to CNS-equivalent zombie systems. These systems, designed to parody the multilevel neuroanatomy of the mammalian CNS, are designed to perform with minimal levels of programmed control. To this point, the best that system components have been able to demonstrate is a tendency to persist in patterns of activation. Despite the limits of current success, their designers postulate that these systems may eventually attain independent human-equivalent consciousness.[15]

## ▷ INTERNET CONSCIOUSNESS

Almost all machine systems have access into the complex, wildly interactive, and minimally controlled system of the Internet. The Internet is now the primary repository of mankind's knowledge, and the largest primary knowledge source available. Assess to this database assists FSM systems in defeating humans at games of intellect. Without access into such an extensive and interconnected knowledge system, complex mathematically based investigations conducted by supercomputers would be working without available data, previous research, and alternative theories. Without Internet access, FSM computer systems operating independently are less likely to provide insights into such complex systems as cosmology, climate, DNA, interface interaction, and central nervous system (CNS) functions.

This data-repository system has its own potential for consciousness. The current complexity of the Internet is difficult to pin down with a concrete number, but it is exceedingly high. Since 1981, the number of Internet-connected systems has been doubling yearly. In the year 2000 there were more than 100 million Internet-connected systems. Today, there are far more Internet-connected PCs than hard-line phone connections.[1] Each PC, each cell phone, each AI, each "super" computer, and each "smart" appliance forms but one of many nodes in this complex system. The Internet is among the most complex of mankind's created artifacts. If the complexity theory of consciousness is correct, it is in such a system that consciousness might arise. The Internet may have already passed the level of complexity attained by the human CNS—the level at which Pierre Teilhard de Chardin proposed that any operational system becomes conscious.[16] The Internet includes within its integrated repertoire a very large store of highly differentiated states of knowledge. Both the database and types of stored knowledge are in the midst of an exponential increase. The Internet is multiscale, often nonlinear, highly heterogeneous, and highly interactive. In biological systems, such a system (the CNS) is utilized to produce thought, cognition, and consciousness. It is postulated that the amount of integrated information that any entity possesses corresponds directly to its level of consciousness. The level of structural "complexity," measured as simultaneous integration and segregation of activity during different states, has been proposed as a potential direct measure of the level of consciousness experienced. The higher the number of connections and the greater the extent of integration in a system, the higher the level of consciousness attainable by the system.[15] If this theory is correct, the Internet integrated with browsers and autonomously operating AI systems is of sufficient complexity and integration to have potential consciousness. Conversely, if current Internet-connected AI multilevel net processing systems are not conscious, complexity $\rightarrow$ consciousness theories may be incorrect.

## INTERNET CAPACITY FOR ASPECTS OF CONSCIOUSNESS

Due to its complexity, the Internet has a greater capacity for intelligence than any single FSM operating as a node in an overall system. Since always on, Internet-based systems have added ability develop established states of focused attention beyond that which can be accomplished by independently operating FSMs that are periodically turned off.[17] Intentionality is tied to hardware, and semantically attributed by humans to the Internet-based search engines that they use.[8] Internal and phenomenological aspects of self-representation can be inferred, based on the capacity for Internet-connected systems to develop and present narratives.[10] It is less clear that any form of volition is within the capacity of these machine systems. However, some authors have begun to discuss volitional aspects of global brain applications that include the Internet.[18] Since the Internet cannot be turned off, the Web as currently designed and developed has considerable autonomy to exist independently of outside controls. The capacities for current self-directed Internet-connected browser systems to perform in these various delineated aspects of consciousness are summarized in Table 13.2.

## INTERFACE CONSCIOUSNESS

At the interface, human consciousness is required. At the interface, the machine system affects and alters human consciousness. Due to the interactive presence of the interface, the human in computer interaction is in a state of consciousness that differs from other nonconnected states of consciousness. At the interface, the interacting computer and the human form an extended mind maintained by the interaction.[19] Such a cognitively interacting "cyborg" differentiates itself from other humans who are not connected to an interface (Fig. 13.1). The cognitive cyborg is a powerful and interesting hybrid, potentially an expert at what can be referred to as dynamical computationalism.[20] As in other areas of computer science, this concept has a philosophic basis. Heidegger argued that we are defined by the experience of our world rather than set apart as a subject directed towards a world of objects.[21] When absorbed in our work, we become part

**Table 13.2** Summary of consciousness criteria with a rating of the capacity for web-based browser systems to meet criteria in each area

| Aspect of consciousness | Web-based browser capacity | |
|---|---|---|
| Intelligence | ++ | Can meet or exceed many of the capabilities of biologic systems |
| Attention | + | Systems exist with the clear capacity for establishing states of focused attention |
| Intention | + | An electronic information paradigm is commonly utilized in the application of programming-based intention in many computer systems |
| Volition | − | To this point, there is little if any test-based evidence that computer systems have developed a capacity for coherent extrapolated volition (CEV) |
| Autonomy | + | Considerable autonomy is possible for Internet-connected programmed browser and robotic systems. These entities are, however, controlled rather than volitionally independent |
| Self-awareness and reflexive consciousness | + | Internal and phenomenological aspects of self-representation can be inferred based on computer-developed and presented narratives |
| Metacognition: Awareness of being aware | − | Metacognitive capacities have not been proven to occur in current interconnected Internet-based systems |
| Evidence for complexity-based consciousness | − | No current evidence indicates the capacity for Web-based browser systems to "rise above programming" |

Rating key: + +, human or supra-human capacity; +, emperic evidence for this capability; −, no emperic evidence for this capability.

of our work (unaware of mouse, keyboard, and joystick) in direct contact with the environment of the cognitive experience.[22] The computer as an external aspect of the environment functions as part of the interfacing human's cognitive processing. The computer scientist Andy Clark and the philosopher David Chambers have joined forces to argue that the human at the interface is part of an extended mind:

*If, as we confront some task, a part of the world functions as a process which, were it to go on in the head, we would have no hesitation in accepting as part of the cognitive process, then that part of the world is (for that time) part of the cognitive process.[23]*

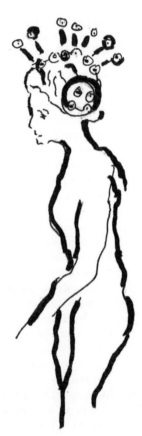

**Figure 13.1** The dreaming cyborg.

At the interface, sensory capacities can be utilized that are beyond the normally interactive human sensorium. At the interface, sight can be parodied and extended beyond the limitations of the sensory organ. Hearing can be augmented, replaced, and extended beyond the biologic infrastructure. New systems incorporating electrophysiologic interactions will extend the interface beyond waking focused consciousness into alternatively conscious states such as dreaming.[24] Emotional expression at the interface can clearly affect the human interaction with the machine system, as well as the interfacing human's emotional relationships with other humans.[25] Humans who spend large amounts of their time at the interface demonstrate changes in their emotional expression, waking mood, and attitude, as well as in their dream content and sleep.[26] At the interface, consciousness is extended and altered for the human. It is somewhat less clear as to how that experience alters and affects the interacting machine.

## SUMMARY: ASPECTS OF MACHINE CONSCIOUSNESS

AI and Web-based search engines meet some of the criteria for having attained human-equivalent aspects of consciousness based on their capabilities in defined aspects of consciousness (intelligence, attention, autonomy, and intention). The high complexity of the Internet provides a potential platform for the development of an independently operating consciousness with complexity theories of consciousness supporting such a capacity to attain conscious function. This question of AI consciousness is no longer hypothetical. The question of AI consciousness has become one of discrimination between forms of machine consciousness and other forms of animal and human consciousness.

At the interface, a new and highly functional form of consciousness is in the process of development. Leibniz's mind-extending calculator has become an extraordinarily powerful tool. Just 30 years ago, few of us spent much of our times at what was then a very limited interface. Now, many of us spend more time at our interface than in any other activity, with the exception, perhaps, for leisure activities.[27] But this interface is still in its developmental infancy. The human/computer cognitive cyborg will define the near future of our species. Unless, of course, the zombie systems come on line with the power of singularity, and we become extraneous.

These forms of machine consciousness are unlike any of the general descriptions of consciousness that have previously been addressed or defined in biologic systems (Chapter 2: The Mechanics of Human Consciousness). They do have overlaps, similarities, and interactions with the other forms of tertiary human-equivalent consciousness. Metacognition and volition, the primary areas of human-equivalent consciousness that have been to this point unattainable by machine systems, are also expressed, in limited fashion, in the sleep-associated states of consciousness that we call dreams.

## Notes

1. Peterson, L., & Davie, B. (2000). *Computer networks: A systems approach* (2nd ed.). San Francisco, CA: Morgan Kaufman Publishers.
2. Bostrom, N. (2014). *Superintelligence: Paths, dangers, strategies*. Oxford: Oxford University Press. Pierre Teilhard de Chardin.
3. Wood, M. (2016). The concept of "cat face": Paul Taylor on machine learning. *London Review of Books, 38*(16), 30–32.
4. Dreyfus, H. (1992). *What computers still can't do*. Cambridge, MA: MIT Press.
5. Li, J., Levine, M. D., An, X., Xu, X., & He, H. (2012). Visual saliency based on scale-space analysis in the frequency domain. *IEEE Transactions on Pattern Analysis and Machine Intelligence, 35*(4), 996–1010.

6. Medalia, A., Aluma, M., Tryon, W., & Merriam, A. (1998). Effectiveness of attention training in schizophrenia. *Schizophrenia Bulletin, 24*(1), 147–152; Sturm, W., Fimm, B., Cantagallo, A., Cremel, N., North, P., Passadori, A., et al. (2003). Specific computerized attention training in stroke and traumatic brain-injured patients. *Zeitschrift fur Neuropsychologie, 14,* 283–292; Wang, T., & Huang, H. (2013). The design and development of a computerized attention-training game system for school age children. In *IADIS international conference e-learning.* Prague, Czech Republic, July 23–26, 2013.

7. Dijksterhuis, A., & Aarts, H. (2010). Goals, attention and (un)consciousness. *Annual Review of Psychology, 61,* 467–490; Lakatos, P., Karmos, G., Mehta, A., Ulbert, I., & Schroeder, C. (2008). Entrainment of neuronal oscillations as a mechanism of attentional selection. *Science, 320,* 110–113; Taylor, J. (2007). Through machine attention to machine consciousness. In A. Chella & R. Manzotti (Eds.), *Artificial consciousness* (pp. 21–47). Charlottesville, VA: Imprint Academic.

8. Pagels, H. R. (1988). *The dreams of reason: The computer and the rise of the sciences of complexity* (pp. 230–232). New York: Bantam Books.

9. Searle, J. (1980). Minds, brains and programs. *The Behavioral and Brain Sciences, 3,* 423.

10. Dennett, D. (1991). *Consciousness explained* (p. 429). Boston, MA: Little, Brown, & Co.

11. Dennett, D. (1981). *Brainstorms: Philosophical essays on mind and psychology* (p. 34). Cambridge, MA: MIT Press.

12. Franklin, S., & Graesser, A. (1997). Is it an agent, or just a program? A taxonomy for autonomous agent. In J. Muller, M. Woodridge, & N. Jennings (Eds.), *Intelligent agents III: Agent theories, architectures and languages* (pp. 21–35). Berlin: Springer.

13. Williams, H. (May, 2012). Why we need "conscious artificial intelligence." Available from http://mindconstruct.com/webpages/newsrec/25. Accessed 23.09.16.

14. Kosko, B. (1993). *Fuzzy thinking: The new science of fuzzy logic* (p. 19). New York: Hyperion.

15. Balduzzi, D., & Tononi, G. (2008). Integrated information in discrete dynamical systems: Motivation and theoretical framework. *PLoS Computational Biology, 4*(6), e1000091; Tononi, G. (2008). Consciousness as integrated information: A provisional manifesto. *Biological Bulletin, 21,* 216–242.

16. de Chardin, P. (1959/1976). *The phenomenon of man.* New York: Harper Perennial.

17. Cho, B., Lee, J., Ku, J., Jang, D., Kim, J., Kim, I., et al. (2002). Attention enhancement system using virtual reality and EEG biofeedback. In *Proceedings of the IEEE Virtual Reality* (pp. 156–163). Los Alamitos, CA: IEEE Computer Society Press.

18. Blackford, R., & Broderick, D. (2014). *Intelligence unbound: The future of uploaded and machine minds.* Chichester: Wiley-Blackwell.

19. Wells, A. (2006). *Rethinking cognitive computation: Turing and the science of the mind.* London: Palgrave.

20. Clark, A. (2008). *Supersizing the mind: Embodiment, action and cognitive extension.* Cambridge, MA: MIT Press.

21. Heidegger, M. (1927). *Being and time.* New York: Harper.

22. Barrett, L. (2011). *Beyond the brain: How body and environment shape animal and human minds* (pp. 149–150). Princeton, NJ: Princeton University Press.

23. Clark, A., & Chambers, D. (1998). The extended mind. *Analysis, 58,* 7–19.

24. Pagel, J. F. (2016). Is the internet conscious? In S. B. Schafer & IGI Global (Eds.), *Exploring the collective unconscious in the age of digital media.* Hershey PA: IGI Global.

25. Darwin, C. (1872/2007). *The expression of the emotions in men and animals.* Mineola, NY: Dover Publications, Inc.; Damasio, A. (1999). *The feeling of what happens: Body and emotion in the making of consciousness.* New York: Harcourt Brace.

26. Gackenback, J., & Kurville, B. (2013). Cognitive structure associated with the lucid features of gamer's dreams. *Dreaming, 23,* 256–267; Stickgold, R. (2000). Tetris dreams: How and when people see pieces from the computer game in their sleep tells of the role dreaming plays in learning. *Scientific American,* October 16. https://www.scientificamerican.com/article/tetris-dreams/. Last accessed 02.11.17. This is a popular summation of Stickgold's series of scientific papers on Tetris.

27. Bureau of Labor Statistics. (2015). *American time use survey.* www.bls.gov/news.release/atus.nr0.htm. Accessed 24.09.16.

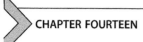

CHAPTER FOURTEEN

# Forms of Machine Dreaming

*And what a strange machine man is. You fill him with bread, wine, fish,
and radishes, and out come sighs, laughter, and dreams.*
**Kazantzakis N. Zorba the Greek.**[1]

Machines can dream. That is to say, machines can meet definition criteria
for dreaming. Machines experience dream-equivalent forms of cognitive
processing. But these dream-equivalent states are not at all the same as
our biological experience of dreaming. These dream states exemplify the
range and particularities of the forms of consciousness. The states of biological dream consciousness are similar to the nonvolitional, nonmeta
forms of consciousness currently exhibited by machine systems. We
humans are the only species that definitely experiences dreaming. We set
the criteria for what we believe is dreaming. We make the definitions.
We develop the technology that defines the tests and the experiments.
We argue the scientific, literary, and social possibilities. We apply our
beliefs and understanding to what dreaming is, and to who or what might
be allowed to have this experience that we call dreaming.

The field of computer science is expanding at an exponential rate. In
this field, applications often take place before philosophy and empiric
understanding can be applied. AI systems and non-human biologic systems display attributes of consciousness. Yet even when it seems logically
apparent we still have no clear definition for consciousness. The question
was once whether such systems were conscious. That question has
morphed into one asking whether or not such systems are developing
human-equivalent aspects of consciousness. And if so, how?

This leads us again to ask—what is human consciousness? What are its
attributes, its functions, and its importance? Consciousness, clearly difficult to globally define, is not one undifferentiated state easy to define or
measure. It is manifest in a multiplicity of states during waking, forms
that differ markedly from one another. The states of consciousness occurring during sleep are so different from states of focused waking that some
neuroscientists argue that dreaming states might be nonconscious.[2] But

*Machine Dreaming and Consciousness.*
DOI: http://dx.doi.org/10.1016/B978-0-12-803720-1.00014-1

how can we say that the cognition of the dreaming states is somehow not reflective of formed consciousness. Dreaming is a ubiquitous human attribute, with well-described functions in the processing of emotions and creativity. These are important functional roles, part of a cognitive process that is preferentially preserved even after extensive brain trauma. Creativity, so tied to dreaming, accounts for our species' success in responding to and profiting from our environment. It seems evident that the presence of dreaming, in any of its myriad forms, is cogent evidence for the presence of consciousness in any system.

## MACHINE DREAM EQUIVALENTS

The ability to achieve dream equivalent processing is already within the capacity of interconnected AI systems. We are in the difficult process of so assessing some systems, such as the Internet; a system that has developed so quickly and with so few controls that it has become somewhat opaque to our understanding. Neural-net and zombie systems in current development, hint at the potential capacity for attaining dream-equivalent states. But they are able to function, at this point in time, at only a minimalistic level. The cyborg interface systems are in some ways the most fascinating, producing what we can view as dyad dream equivalence—a state of dreaming shared between human and machines.

## MACHINE DREAMS—MESSAGES FROM GOD

Computers routinely access their programmed operative instructions. Many computer systems are interactive with the operator. This sentence is being typed into a writing system on a personal computer, and as such, in interacting with my computer I am supplying information and exerting control. And while I am not changing basic programming language, I am affecting and manipulating program expression. This interaction with my computer is as if it were from an interactive creator. A machine controller might be viewed from the machine perspective as an interactive god. So defined as a message from the controller, accessible programmed information can be considered a form of dreaming

(dreaming defined as a message from god). Humans strive diligently for such contact with their gods. As based on level of access, computers are far closer to their controllers than most humans.

## MACHINE DREAMS—SLEEP-ASSOCIATED MENTATION

Independent, solitary, finite state machines (FSMs) do not possess the processing ability within their strictly defined states to support a logical analogue for sleep. And since they have no sleep analogue, they should not be able to experience dreaming sleep—defined as sleep-associated mentation. During designated sleep modes in an FSM, the machine is actually turned off except when responding to a timed cyclical self-monitoring program that turns the machine on, makes assessments of machine status, and/or runs alternative programming (e.g., the SETI project), and then shuts it down, or when indicated applies protective programming.[3] It has been proposed that dream-equivalent processing occurs during sleep mode activity in computer systems. In biologic systems this perspective has been extended into the proposal that dreams might function in defragmentation and system cleaning removing unneeded, cluttered, and useless waking data from consciousness. It is suggested that it is this process that contributes to the perceived "degraded and/or degenerative" (nonlogical) aspects of the dream state.[4] Assuming such a perspective has led some to the belief that dreams include meaningless content and lack other functions.[5]

Finite state machines are always, however, in one defined state—either on or off. This difference between machine sleep (off) and biologic sleep (on) denotes a profound difference between biologically based and machine systems. As Descartes suggested centuries ago, there is little evidence that an off-state equivalent is possible for any biologic system that is actually alive.[6]

Yet in a system such as the Worldwide Web in which finite state machines serve as interconnected nodes within an extended system, a form of active sleep can occur. Independent of individual nodes dropping out or being turned off, the system as a whole is always on, maintained in a variable on-mode of interconnected data flow. The periods of low data flow in such a multiplex interconnected system correspond to the human sleep cycle, when less interactive operator activity is taking place. These periods of low activity can be viewed as periods of "Internet sleep." During these Internet sleep periods a large amount of complex processing can take place.

This activity is often unapparent at the computer interface and not available in the next wake period without probing or applied analysis. During such Internet equivalent sleep periods, the system as a whole resets, recharges, and achieves an equilibrium that is more difficult to achieve during the high-flow wake data periods. Internet sleep, like human sleep, is a highly complex, highly differentiated, and highly integrated state. The cognitive processing occurring during Internet sleep meets axis criteria for dreaming in that it occurs during a state that can be defined as sleep, is available as a report at the interface, and includes interpretable content. During such system sleep, exceedingly complex processing produces a lower error rate than processing that takes place during congested periods. During system sleep periods, systems operate closer to optimal performance than during wake periods of high data flow and congestion.[7] This sleep-associated cognitive processing can be viewed as a state of machine-equivalent dreaming. This form of machine dreaming has far more similarities with biologic dream states than the "screensaver" modes previously proposed as computer-based equivalents for dreaming.[4]

## MACHINE DREAMS—METAPHOR

The most common definition of dream is loosely Freudian, what you will find if you Google or search the index at your local library. Metaphors of wish fulfillment abound: dream marriages, dream vacations, dream homes, dream sex, and dream cars. The Internet has become a repository for such human dreams, the site where we search for patterns that reflect and perhaps even consummate our dreams. Some of this search we define by our own actions, but much of what we end up exploring is based on the structure of the Internet, our access systems, the alignment of the search engine that we use, and the slant of the programming applied by outside sources (note the commercial importance of highlighting on the first page of a Google search). We fill the Internet with our metaphors of dream. That material, our best visual and literary attempts at describing our dreams, differs minimally from a reported dream (some are actually dream reports). If you ask a search engine for a dream, this is what you will be shown. These reports meet criteria for dreaming, yet they are the reports, the results, of dreaming in a biologic system. They are not an ongoing real-time component of an actual machine process of dreaming. In searching for and reporting a dream on the Internet you might obtain reports of biologic dreams. Or a defined goal can be set for that which meets criteria as a computer-generated dream.[8] Such an Internet dream can be viewed as another layer of metaphor, or from the computer standpoint, as a searchable database of human dream equivalents.

## MACHINE DREAMS—BIZARRE & ALTERNATIVE OUTCOMES

Artificial neural networks incorporate on—off processing, multiple connections, multiple levels, and dynamic feedback that takes place in temporal sequence or in artificial pseudo-time space. These systems attempt to parody physiological aspects of biologic neural-net processing. Neural equivalent processes of associative, multilevel memory, and cognitive feedback are incorporated into these systems that approximate similar fundamental components of the states of biologic dreaming. Neural network AI systems can be trained to respond and adjust to changing stimuli in order to accomplish programmed goals. Entry into and exit from any specific fuzzy state is approximate. As in dreaming, there is the possibility that autonomous states will be created that reflect alternative state transition to new, unexpected sets of solutions.

Neural network hardware processing produces outcomes that can be considered as indeterminate or hallucinatory. Confused or logically unusable real number stimuli, noise, and partial or incomplete training make AI machine dysfunction increasingly probable as systems become larger and artificial neural density increases. At least 3/8 of the results obtained from simple system neural network processing can be viewed as indeterminate, noncontributory, or hallucinatory.[9] These results can be viewed as evidence for machine dysfunction, hypothetical and nonapplicable to real-world situations. Such "degraded mentation" can be viewed as a form of machine dreaming.

Learning-trained AI systems are designed to produce goal-reflective results that have continuity with the problem presented. But sometimes the answer produced by these systems is as diffuse and imprecise as any biologic and interactively psychoanalyzed dream. These results can be, however, potentially useful alternative views of the problem presented and the systems' experience of its own external reality. Goal-defined systems are likely to reject such alternative analyzands assuring that results "outside-the—box" will not be considered or included in the analysis. Goal-defined result interpretation and applied operator control limits system creativity and the capacity for that system to produce alternative responses. It is very possible that the inclusion of alternative outcomes may be required if a logically programmed system is ever to develop the capacity to function in a sometimes illogical human-described and -defined world, where flexible, alternative approaches are required and sometimes the norm. The integration of dream-like alternative processing offers the possibility that such systems might be better able to interrelate with humans. It is also possible that through incorporating such machine dreaming equivalents, machines might develop further capacities for human-like dream functioning, such as in creativity.

Psychoanalysts define dreaming as bizarre/hallucinatory mentation. Through the Web our systems access exceedingly bizarre material, some stranger than we might have believed possible. Some of that material is just strange. Other material is the result of exceedingly complex programming and processing. An approach such as weather/climate forecasting will incorporate and integrate a series of mathematical models constructed around extended sets of dynamic equations that are impossible to solve through analytical methods. The accuracy of the results and predictions of analysands varies with the density and quality of data, as well as any deficiencies and limitations inherent in the numerical models. The outcomes derived are sometimes unexpected and often difficult to explain. Important contributory data may be bottlenecked, corrupted, or lost, and the complexly developed analysis that results may provide unexpected and alternative answers to questions that the observer is unsure how even to ask. Such results share characteristics with dreaming: an integration of extensive sensory data; the associative interactions of many memory processing subsystems; variable memory access; attained results that diverge from expectations and are often incomprehensible except when presented as a time-based visual display; and result analysis, that like dream interpretation is often a metaphoric and allegoric process affected by the training and belief systems of the researchers. Such a dynamic analysis approximates on almost every level the process and concept of a bizarre and hallucinatory dream.

## MACHINE DREAMS—THE PHENOMENOLOGY

Dream phenomena—the images, emotions, and associated memories that we typically associate with dreams—have continuity with our life experience. Despite their ubiquity, each dream is uniquely individual and tells an emotional, complex, and continually changing story. Dream emotions are most often negative.[10] This characteristic is particularly evident when the dream is part of the process of integrating emotion and trauma. After trauma, bad dreams can become nightmares.

Computer systems work with data representations amalgamated into words, narrative, emotions, and visual images. The Internet is an archive of our hopes, our indiscretions, the images of our successes and failures, and our dreams and nightmares—both real and in metaphor. In searching and using the Internet, AI systems are utilizing this human-based content data set. IBM's Watson is a strongly interactive web browser with self-learning capacity as well as a capacity for emotional expression (Watson is programmed to produce positive imagery that goes well beyond the Imoge of a smiley face). While attempts have been made to set performance boundaries and defining algorithms, Watson's software built on 720 processor cores running in parallel, can frequently produce nonsense, if interesting, answers to queries made outside specific areas of defined expertise. Such responses can be construed to indicate the limits of conscious and nonconscious functioning for such a system.[11] These systems can utilize the Internet data set as well as their own data history and processing to create a variably excluded set that includes imprecise data. Such indeterminate and hallucinatory data, integrated with human-defined dream reports, can be used to produce remarkably diffuse imagery that has dream-like phenomenology. These images have continuity with waking experience. They are visually unique, complex, and constantly changing. Some human viewers consider these images to be aesthetically pleasing. Some have the capacity to induce emotional reactions in the viewer. Google refers to these images as AI dreams.[8]

## ARTIFICALLY CREATED REM SLEEP

At this point it is unclear what cognitive capacities might be attainable by neural net-based neuroanatomic and perfect zombie systems. Such systems are designed to approximate human-equivalent complexity using artificial neuron hardware. As based on complexity > consciousness theory, such systems built with human-derived components have the potential for attaining independently functioning human-equivalent consciousness. Of course, these are unproven theories and this is far from a surety. It is also possible that these systems may have little more capability than the ability to glow in the dark.

Machine learning AI, and networking systemically designed to produce alternative, indeterminate, and/or hallucinatory data analysis will be integrated into these systems. It is possible that such autonomously functioning and minimally controlled systems will independently develop complex processing states such as REM sleep. This, of course, would indicate their capacity to meet even another definition level for dream equivalence. It would also, however, indicate their capacity for high level of self-organization including the capacity to develop human-equivalent physiologic states that we do not clearly understand. The designers of these systems postulate that forms of cognitive processing will develop independently of operator input. Such a system might has the potential for developing fully human-equivalent consciousness.

But today, it remains debatable as to whether the zombie systems will have any capacity for consciousness. If such a breakthrough does occur, in order for these systems to develop forms of human-like consciousness, such zombies might require the capacity to dream. It is possible that during dream-equivalent states such a system could potentially become lucid, entering a state of consciousness in which it attains and exerts control of potential outcomes and starts to control its own story. This would be the machine equivalent of lucid dreaming: a state of dream-like consciousness during which the system would be capable of the machine-equivalent behavior of reaching out and pushing buttons. Such a lucid system would be able to independently change and control its data flow. Such a lucid system would unquestionably be conscious.

## MACHINE-CREATED DREAMS

Humans in their art, their writing, and their films have concentrated on developing their ability to create artificially produced dreams. This is particularly true of filmmaking, a technical process that incorporates images, acted emotions, and sounds into a narrative structure. This process lends itself to artificial simulation. In creating a film, the filmmaker artificially approximates many of the same biological systems incorporated cognitively into dreams. There is little question that AI systems can create simulacrum interface dreamscapes that include similar visual, memory, and emotional components to those that comprise a biologic dream.

The limitations of this process are not technical. The limitations are based on our limited human understanding of the dream states. Reported dreams in their most basic forms describe the way that we organize experience. While complex, the technical paradigms of this process can be artificially constructed. In our viewing or reading of constructed dreams, we interject our own memories, emotions, and imagery into the experience. And once so enmeshed, the human or the machine filmmaker can entice us into a vicarious experience of mental images that resemble less a dream and more the vivacity of actual experience. This capability is well within the capacity of computer-based systems. Such an increased level of machine-integrated presentation will be required if interface interactions with humans are to develop in a direction that can be considered positive for both the human and machine. In order to better interact machine systems must incorporate the way that humans organize experience. The interactive presentation at the interface closely resembles what might be best described as a projected dream.

## MACHINE DREAMS AT THE HUMAN INTERFACE

We are spending more and more of our waking time within this bidirectional machine interface. Today our children and our mates often spend more time interfacing with their extending machines than they do in interacting each other and with us. New interface systems under current development will reach beyond the sensory modalities that we utilize in our waking environmental interactions to include nonsensory modalities such as frequency-based physiologic electrical fields. In the near future, cognitive systems utilized in meditation, sleep, and dream states will become part of our interface interaction.

The human enmeshed within such a system will have an even greater opportunity to develop and expand capacities as a cognitive cyborg. This is already the case in our most complex systems such as our planes, exploration, and weapon systems. The interfaced human and the attached machine become something larger, smarter, and potentially more interesting than either system when disconnected. Today's gamers, sometimes seeming to inhabit an alternative universe, are limited by the current technology of sensory interface systems. But even so, their interface expe-rience extends into their dreaming, so that after spending waking time at the interface, their waking thoughts, their sleep, and their dream contents are altered.[12] The interface interaction also affects the machine, changing associated memories (data histories), and extending the development of interactive machine/human dream equivalents. We humans have incorpo-rated our memories, or visions, and our dreams into the available data stream. The machine, pushed to capacity in its attempts to utilize and integrate all available data in the attempt to approximate the set goals that we have defined, will utilize all pertinent (and even nonpertinent) data. Bidirectionally, the system using these data has continuity with the dream consciousness of the involved human. The resulting human—machine interaction can become a sometimes confusing, hallucinatory, and crea-tively interactive dream-like, dream-equivalent state. Humans when con-fronted with dreams are likely, as David Foulks has so kindly pointed out, to "prematurely forsake the possibility of disciplined empirical analysis."[13] We should expect no less from our interface partners when they are con-fronted with dream-equivalent states that include bizarre-hallucinatory metaphors, novel visual imagery, and unexpected data streams of memory. At the interface, the cognitive cyborg is dreaming.

## MACHINE DREAMING—SYSTEM SUMMARY AND COMPARISON

Computer systems are becoming increasingly complex as they incorporat alternative logic hardware, programming software, and extended interfaces into their systems. Computer scientists are not using this approach in order to help their systems to dream. They are using these approaches because of the limits of systems that utilize only strict, controlled logic in their functions. Such predicate logic systems have had significant difficulty functioning in the common sense and difficult to log-ically understand human interactive environment. Many humans have similar if opposite difficulties in their attempts to interact and function with concrete machine logics that often require a yes/no answer to ques-tions that appear from the human perspective to be complex and diffuse. In any somewhat illogical environment, humans are able to comfortably operate without a theory of mind. AI systems are being created that can better approach the external environment in ways similar to the commonsense approaches used by humans. Such a change in processing requires the ability to utilize and process alternative outcomes that may be inconsistent with concrete logic. This process is to some degree controllable using programmed rules, goal setting, result interpretation and winnowing. But increasingly such systems are being designed with hardware and software that operate outside controller purview.

Alternative cognitive processing has dream-equivalence—these forms of consciousness different from focused waking, are not fully volitional, and sometimes produce apparently illogical and difficult to interpret outcomes (Table 14.1). Isolated finite state machines built with predicate, concrete logic programming, such as the typical personal computer, have limited capacities for achieving defined dream equivalence. These systems can have interface interactions that produce a shared dream-like cognitive experience. This capacity will increase as interface systems incorporate expanded sensory and nonsensory extenders. Extension of FSM software processing capacity into areas of approximate or fuzzy logic can be utilized to extend system capacity beyond concrete logic applications, while increasing the possibility of alternative and/or unexpected outcomes.

Internet connection allows for expansion beyond the individual FSM into areas where the FSM (PC or cell) is but an access node in an overall operating system that is never turned off. Such a system has periods of high and low data flow with the periods of low flow corresponding to human sleep times. Such periods are a machine form of active sleep. The Internet also offers access to an extended database of human dream metaphors and memories. The addition of AI self-teaching (learning) capacity to a neural-net hardware and software format increases the likelihood that indeterminate, hallucinatory, alternative, and unexpected results will be produced by the system.

AI systems are extending their capacity for meeting the various defined criteria for dream-like mentation. Many current systems have the capacity to develop dream-like or dream-equivalent cognitive processing. This goal is not routinely stated and is in many cases not understood as an objective by the programmers and theorists involved in the process. But current predicate logic systems have clear limitations, and there is an obvious need for developing systems with greater anthropomorphic capacity, able to integrate and interact better with humans in the same manner that humans interact with one another. There is evidence suggesting that such systems function better in the commonsense-based

Table 14.1 Machine cognitive processing types—Capacity for meeting dream definition criteria

| | Sleep mentation | Dream metaphor mentation | Bizarre, hallucinatory mentation | Dream phenomenology and human memory access | Dream-like mentation interface capacity |
|---|---|---|---|---|---|
| Solitary finite state machine (FSM) | − | − | − | − | + |
| Solitary FSM with self-learning and neural net programming | − | − | ++ | ++ | ++ |
| Nodal FSM Internet connected | − | ++ | − | + | + |
| Internet-connected FSM with fuzzy logic capacity | − | ++ | + | ++ | + |
| Global Internet with browser connection | ++ | ++ | + | ++ | + |
| Internet-connected AI system with learning capacity | ++ | ++ | + | ++ | ++ |
| Internet-connected neural network-based AI | ++ | ++ | +++ | ++ | ++ |
| Neuroanatomic–based zombie system | ? | ? | +++ | − | + |
| Perfect zombie system | ? | ? | ++ | − | +++ |

Key: − , none; ?, unknown; + , ++, ++ +, accessed criteria compliance.

human environment than systems limited to predicate logic.[14] During sleep-like states of low data flow, error rates decline and system function improves.[7] Extending system processing capacity beyond the constraints of predicate logic can improve system processing capacity in specific areas such as scheduling and adaptable goal attainment.[15] And it is becoming apparent that such flexible logic systems are required as a component of Internet browsing systems if such systems are to be congruent with human-based requirements for commonsense data access. These systems have the ability to represent and process human metaphor, bringing together and interconnecting stored human visual and text-based memories into narrative stories that have the characteristics of dreaming mentation. Neural-net systems have the capacity to go even further, bringing indeterminate and/or hallucinatory results into the resultant response paradigm. Visually presented, results can even look like dreamscapes.[8] The processed results presented by systems such as IBM's Watson include emotional cues in the attempt to positively improve the interface interaction.[16] The process of interaction at the interface then becomes even more dream-like as it includes all the basic phenomenological structures typical of dreaming: bidirectional visual imagery, associative memories, and emotions.

In the near future, computer systems will extend their presentation capacity at the interface into creating film-like artificial dreams. The technical processes of filmmaking are well within the capacity of AI systems. Interface systems are already starting to incorporate aspects of the nonsensory electrophysiological systems that are predominately active during dreaming and dream-like waking states. The human interacting with such a system is likely to experience an amplification of the dream-like aspects of the cognitive cyborg states. Independently organized zombie systems are being developed. If functional, such systems may have the potential for autonomous, volitional consciousness. Since such systems are being designed as closely as currently possible on human physiology, these systems may develop similarly organized physiologic states (e.g., REM sleep). In order to function as human in the human-defined world, these systems are likely to require the ability to experience human-equivalent dreaming. As based on what we understand of human dreaming, the human-equivalent machine dream marking this reach beyond programing might include an image like that depicted on the cover of this book.

# Notes

1. Kazantzakis, N. (1946/2012). *Zorba the Greek*. New York: Simon and Schuster.
2. Crick, F., & Koch, C. (1992). The problem of consciousness. *Scientific American, 267*, 152–159.
3. Participate in SETI@home https://setiathome.berkeley.edu/sah_participate.php. Accessed 10.10.16.
4. Crick, F., & Mitchenson, G. (1983). The function of dream sleep. *Nature, 304*, 111–114.
5. Hobson, J. A. (1996). *Consciousness*. New York: Scientific American Library.
6. Descartes, R. (1641). Objections against the meditations and replies. In J. M. Adler (Ed-in chief), *Great books of the Western world: Bacon, Spinoza and Descartes (1993)*. Chicago, IL: Encyclopedia Britannica Inc.
7. Peterson, L., & Davie, B. (2000). *Computer networks: A systems approach* (2nd ed.). San Francisco, CA: Morgan Kaufman Publishers.
8. Google's AI can dream, and here's what it looks like. *IFLScience*. www.iflscience.com/technology/artificial-intelligence-dream. Accessed 13.09.16.
9. Gillies, D. (1996). *Artificial intelligence and the scientific method*. Oxford: Oxford University Press.
10. Kramer, M. (2007). *The dream experience: A system exploration*. New York: Routledge.
11. Baker, S. (2011). *"Watson" has serious limitations*. triblive.com/x/pittsburghtrib/opinion/.../s_723648.html Accessed 10.10.16. Most of the available information on the new GOOGLE and IBM systems is provided in press releases and popular blurbs that have been released by the companies.
12. Gackenback, J., & Kurville, B. (2013). Cognitive structure associated with the lucid features of gamer's dreams. *Dreaming, 23*, 256–267; Stickgold, R. (2000). Tetris dreams: How and when people see pieces from the computer game in their sleep tells of the role dreaming plays in learning. *Scientific American*, October 16.
13. Foulks, D. (1985). *Dreaming: A cognitive-psychological analysis*. Hillsdale, NJ: Lawrence-Erlbaum Associates.
14. Barrat, J. (2013). *Our final invention: Artificial intelligence and the end of the human era*. New York: Thomas Dunne Books.
15. Kosko, B. (1993). *Fuzzy thinking: The new science of fuzzy logic*. New York: Hyperion.
16. Ewbank, K. (2016). *IBM's Watson gets sensitive*. www.i-programmer.info/news/105-artificial.../9477-ibms-watson-gets-sensitive.htm. Accessed 10.10.16.

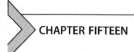

# CHAPTER FIFTEEN

# The Antropomorphic Dream Machine

*And if he were forcibly dragged up the steep and rugged ascent of the cave and not let go till he had been dragged out into the sunlight, would he not experience pain, and so struggle against this? And would he not, as soon as he emerged into the light, his eyes dazzled, be unable to see any of the things he was now told were unhidden?*

**Plato—The Cave: The Third Stage.[1]**

*We can consider our universe filled with clocks, equations and science as much as with dreams memories and laughter.*

**Canales J. (2015). The Physicist and the Philosopher.[2]**

The human species is fascinated by dreams. Dreams are part and parcel of our earliest recorded history, defining and reflecting our religious beliefs, our art, our science, our creativity, and our possibilities for the future. Six thousand years ago, in some of the first recorded scripts, King Gudea sent copies of his dream out into the ancient world. In our era, another King, who using spell-binding rhetoric, moved us to understand and believe in the possibility of change, repeating over and over, "I have a dream."[3] Dreams are illuminated through literature and song. Dreams are intimate, often shared in courtships and relationship building. Dream sharing plays an integral role in friendship and social discovery.[4] As individuals and societies, most all of us use our dreams.[5]

In the psychoanalytic era, it seemed that dreams might be a window into understanding the reasons and the malapropisms accounting for our species' behaviors. But psychoanalysis failed when applied to medicine, psychiatry, and neuroscience. It turned out to be a perspective based far more on belief than evidence. The unfortunate sequels to the psychoanalytic era included perceived shame, requirements for expensive and prolonged one-on-one therapy, and long-term seclusion of psychiatric patients into warehouse environments providing minimal, even dysfunctional care.[6] Some of the failure of psychoanalysis was reflected onto

*Machine Dreaming and Consciousness.*
DOI: http://dx.doi.org/10.1016/B978-0-12-803720-1.00015-3

dreaming. Dream interpretation was dismissed as psuedoscience, and dreaming de-emphasized.

Today, computer programmers and theorists expend considerable effort, resources, and money in the attempt to develop alternative processing approaches that improve machine ability to function and interact with humans. This requirement to develop a commonsense (sometimes illogical) human interaction has led them to develop forms of processing in their systems that, based on definition and phenomenology, meet criteria as forms of consciousness and dream. At this point in time it is as somewhat unclear for machines, as it is for humans, what this capacity for dream-equivalent processing portends.

# HUMAN DREAMS

Most humans have no difficulty in experiencing dream consciousness. On average, we wake at least twice a week with unexpected memories, vivid images, and intense emotions, all part of the narratives that we call dreams. Many of us experience and remember far more. We often use the dreams that we remember in our decision making, in developing our attitudes towards ourselves and others, in relationships, in planning our future, in our work and play, and in our creative process.[5]

The capacity to dream characterizes our species. We do not know if any other species has the capacity to dream. From in the distant past, the time of the Paleolithic cave paintings, our species has adapted and changed more readily than any other.[7] Our ability to dream contributes to our ability to explore alternative approaches and our adaptability in developing new ones. As such, our ability to dream is a component of the basic cognitive framework that has assisted our species in becoming ascendant and dominant on this planet. Yet in today's world, we typically dismiss, ignore, and scientifically denigrate both our own dreams, and our capacity as humans to dream. We are investing great effort, insight, and resources into developing the capacity for our machines to achieve dream-equivalent consciousness. Strangely, we invest next to nothing into attempts to understand the dynamics and science behind our human capacity to dream.

## HUMAN INTEREST IN DREAMING

While the fields of AI and robotics are pushing for more flexible and dream-like programming, the study of dreams in humans and other biologic systems has gone in another direction. This current period of reassessment reflects a nadir of scientific interest. In a search of Pubmed, the primary index of published scientific and medical research, the percentage of research and review papers addressing the topic of dreams has dropped markedly in the last 15 years.[8] This decrease in interest in dreaming reflects the change in focus from dream-based psychoanalysis to the presumed physiologically equivalent state of REM sleep. Fifty years ago, we thought we knew far more about dreaming than about sleep. Psychoanalysis and the REM sleep = dreaming equation generated a huge amount of dream research and literature. In the US, almost all research monies ear-marked for the study of sleeping consciousness (dreaming) ended up going to programs that studied REM sleep in lab animals. Today, there are many researchers trained in techniques and active in the study of REM sleep, yet there are very few with the background, interest, or money that can be applied to the study of biologic dreaming. Just decades ago, the major sleep research societies dedicated sections and entire tracts of study to dreaming. Today, the major sleep research meeting (2016 APSS) had more than 1200 abstracts posted pertaining to the fields of sleep study. Only three addressed dream. Most philosophers, psychologists, and physicians have moved on to other topics. Across the fields of neuroscience, the cognitive states of dream consciousness are rarely addressed.

It is difficult to determine whether the level of interest in dreaming might be declining for the general population. Books on dreaming, particularly on the topic of dream interpretation, have always been popular. The second book printed on Guttenberg's press, after the Bible, was an index of dream symbols, titled Oneiromancy.[9] Such books are still being published, but today, less often than how-to books on sleep topics like insomnia. Perhaps, human interest in dreaming is less pronounced than in past eras. Note the initial quote in this chapter from Plato's Cave.[1] It has been over 2000 years since Plato described a basic human impulse to risk even blindness in order to escape from the darkness and uncertainty of dream.

As noted in this book, there are multiple approaches to hardware, software, and systems for creating artificial machine-based constructs of consciousness. Frustrated in their attempts to create AI and robotic systems able to coherently function in the commonsense world of humanity, computer scientists have pushed beyond the constraints of concrete logic to create systems that have the capacity for fuzzy, alternative, and even irrational logic. In order to assist their machines in functioning in the human world, a world that may not have a logical theory of mind, they have had to incorporate less controlled and less defined cognitive processing. Some of this processing cognitively approximates the biologic processes of dreaming. In order to better interface with humans, computer systems are being programmed with the capacity to artificially create these dream-like states. At the human–machine interface, bidirectional systems are being designed to have an expanded capacity to interact with humans in dream and dream-like states of consciousness, using dream-associated sensory and nonsensory interface modalities.

This leads to the interesting conundrum in which computer scientists, rather than neuroscientists or psychiatrists, have assumed the role of today's experts on the cognitive states of dreaming and dream equivalence. These theorists have an uncertain advantage in that they know very little about the biologic state of dreaming, its history, or the prior constructs of presumed understanding. Yet the systems they are creating now have the capacity to meet or approximate criteria for each of the primary definitions that we use for dreaming. These systems share with humans forms of cognitive processing that have characteristic dream phenomenology. As based on definition, functioning, and associated characteristics, these systems are capable of dream-equivalent states. Yet there are still some definition criteria that remain beyond the capacity of our artificial creations. These are primarily those that cannot be compared or tested—those primarily based on human belief and metaphor—what Nietzsche described as truth:

> a movable host of metaphors, metonymies, and anthropomorphisms: in short, a sum of human relations which have been poetically and rhetorically intensified, transferred and embellished, and which after long usage, seem to people to be fixed, canonical, and binding.[10]

Despite such anthropomorphic defensive logistics, viewed from within the rational context presented in this book, we humans have given our machines the capacity to dream. Today, machines can meet criteria in part or in form for every definition that our species has developed for dreaming. But these machine dreams are not what we may have come to expect. They differ markedly from the fantasies portrayed in sci-fi films and fictions. Machine dream-equivalents are those machine-based dream-like forms of cognitive processing that meet our human-based criteria for dreaming. The exception is the anthropocentric definition. If only humans can dream, the machine's potential for meeting that definition rests fully in its potential to attain and maintain the pretence of being human. That is the only way for a machine to encompass an anthropomorphic exclusive definition, stating that only humans have the capacity to dream. For some, it is frightening and offensive to postulate this capacity for our artificially created machines. But a machine operates best when programmed to attain set goals, such as the ability to fully mimic human appearance and behavior. At some point there may be no way to tell which creature is human and which machine. This has been suggested as the point at which machines will fully meet criteria for human-equivalent consciousness.[11]

## CYBORG DREAMING

We spend a large amount of time interfaced with our machines. That interaction extends beyond that time of actual contact. Later in wake and in our sleep, in day and night, our dreams are of experiences at the interface.[12] Sensory augmentation and new approaches to access are bringing to the interface the nonsensory physiologic systems that we typically use in alternative states of consciousness. Such systems will allow us to further develop the experience of shared dream-like cognition— augmenting our capacity for dream-like cognitive states such as default mind-wandering, day-dreaming, creativity, and states of focused and unfocused meditation.[8] We have been trained to accept such experience when learning to view and interact with film screen illusion and reality. Only, this interaction will have tighter suture, providing an even more intense alternative to the often profound experience of watching a film. The interactive bidirectional interface denotes an alternative state of consciousness that is shared between human and machine. This is the domain of the dreaming cyborg (Fig. 13.1)—part human, part machine, enmeshed and sutured into shared experience.

In the last half of the 20th century, we have used the computer to extend our human capacities in remarkable ways. Our mathematical capacities and approaches have changed and expanded. Shortcuts and approximations (remembering the slide rule) are rarely required. What were formerly burdensome and sometimes impossible summations can now be quickly accomplished. Computer-controlled robotic systems have extended our perceptual and operational capacities into the exploration of outer space. We are able to collect and maintain a database of records documenting our most trivial interactions and accomplishments. We use computer systems to search through this collected cloud of debris for nuggets of insight. We use them to process, edit, translate, and disseminate our findings. We have access to an Internet database of knowledge that is far beyond the capacity of any autodidactic human or record-keeping library. We use our computers in research, in politics, in social interactions, and in gaming to keep us occupied and entertained. As replacement for human contact, these interactions can help in keeping us from feeling isolated and alone.

The dreaming human/machine cyborg has the potential to achieve cognitive breakthroughs that have up until this point been impossible for either system to achieve in isolation. The machine offers computational capacity, extended perceptions, data access, integrative, and presentational capacity beyond the capacity of any human. The human supplies the ability to interpret data without the need for a logical theory of mind. The human, with the ability to function seamlessly in a commonsense world, within the interface, has the capacity to escape into, if not conquer, virtual worlds. Working in concert with artificial systems, we can solve difficult and seemingly intractable problems. But there is little evidence that the interface with these systems has made individual humans more intelligent. As artificial systems progress in both complexity and capabilty, our capacities remain much the same. Our machines, our artificial creations, are undergoing an exponential increase in intelligence, in perceptual capacity, in their ability to expand aspects of consciousness, and in their development of additional interface interactions. Tied to an inherently conservative and slowly changing biology, independently functioning humans continue to work from within the same structurally limited framework. Yet in the dyad, it is the human who has the role of attempting to globally understand problems and set appropriate goals. Humans are still the ones with the capacity to metaphysically comprehend the potential results of behaviors. But that is not to say that humans cogently use such capacities. Human behaviors can be remarkably stupid, ill-considered, and self-destructive. In the dyad, it is the human who brings a capacity for metaphysics, insight, and conscience to the table. Dependent on humans for such values, it is doubtful that human—machine cyborgs will behave in any better fashion than humans operating independently.

Today, when humans enter into intellectual competitions with machine systems, they rarely win. Yet at this point in time, AI has yet to achieve some fully human-equivalent capacities for mental cognition. Among these unattained human capacities is the ability to fully produce a cognitively equivalent state of dreaming. While computers, AI systems, and neural nets can achieve a variety of the dream-equivalent mental states, none of these states fully approximate to the human dream. AI robotic systems, in order to function, must have self-awareness and conti-nuity within their experienced environment, as well as the ability to learn in response to environmental change. In order to function in the human commonsense world with its limited theory of mind, these systems require an ability to function and process using techniques extending beyond the limits of parametric logic. But AI systems still lack dream-associated aspects of self-awareness, intentionality, independent volition, and autonomy independent of programming. Independent of human pro-grammers and their human interface, our AI systems, our neural nets, and even our zombies have little, if any, capacity to function outside the tightly defined logics we have programmed. There is little evidence that in any of their current forms, these systems have been able to rise above our programming. There are many levels of metaphysical consciousness and conscience that machines have yet to explore. There are many levels of creative, artistic, and integrative capacity they have yet to attain.

## THESE ARE NOT DREAMS

This is an exciting time. We are giving the capacity to dream to our machines. We may have only limited understanding of dreaming, but we have the capacity to artificially create its equivalent cognition for our artificial creations. This capacity, even in current limited forms, is profoundly changing how these systems operate. Artificial systems programmed with parametric concrete logic have been incredibly useful, but these systems require the assistance of humans in order to function in the human environment. Neural net systems and fuzzy logic robots are already demonstrating an increased capacity for operating in a more commonsense, human-like fashion. But these systems are still in their infancy. In order to more fully integrate into the human world, these systems will require even greater human-like capacities. They will explore alternative and illogical outcomes, in hopes that they will be better able to develop creative resolutions for complex problems. In this journey, zombie systems may develop dream-associated physiologic states, perhaps even conscience, and metaphysical views of their universe that will include a persisting role for humans. But today, we have no concept as to how this might occur.

At the interface, we are interacting and learning in concert with our machines. There seems a clear logic that we should at least try to understand this combined journey, as this process of change affects both systems. Our future will include human—machine cognitive cyborg dyads dreaming in concert. We can only hope that the outcomes will be positive. These dyads have the potential to be extraordinarily creative and/or extraordinarily confused. In the future, they will have much greater capability than today's drone pilots. Like those enmeshed pilots, they will have the potential to be extraordinarily destructive.

Our future will include autonomous robots with the capacity to assist us in operating in our commonsense human world. In order to do this, these systems will have some form of the human-equivalent capacity to respond to illogical situations in which there is no apparent theory of mind. In order to create such systems, current controls of tightly programmed logic will be discarded. The operations of such a system will no longer be apparent to either the programmer or the interactive operator. Some of the results of that processing will be illogical and hallucinatory and, like human dreaming, will be sometimes ignored yet often utilized.

Our future will include neuroanatomic and perfect zombie systems. Multilayered neural net systems embedded in chemical baths and initiated with an electrical impulse have already demonstrated de novo neural equivalent firing activity.[13] Governments and private sector billionaires are investing millions of dollars and immense effort into the creation of such systems. In the next 20 years, multiple versions will come on line. Major results are possible. The expectations are huge.

## DREAMING AS A MARKER FOR HUMANITY: THE ARGUMENT FOR HUMAN DREAMING

Beyond REM sleep, dream recall frequency is the only characteristic of dreaming that has been studied in scientific depth. Dream content is affected by a huge number of conflicting variables that are difficult to methodologically control. With computer assistance, we have the ability to control for transference, report expectations, and researcher bias (continuity has proven an exceptionally difficult variable). Such a controlled methodological approach requires considerable effort, and few aspects of dream content have been studied. In this era dream research receives minimal funding. Dream use and dream incorporation into waking behavior are easily accessible, but in today's world scientific research is almost entirely dependent on government and/or pharmacological funding. Since such studies have never been funded, little supports research interest. Dream research is funded, at some level, in Canada, the United Kingdom, the Netherlands, Germany, Austria, and Finland. In the United States a limited support is applied primarily to the treatment of nightmares in patients with PTSD. PTSD is a modern, social, and politically developed epidemic with disordered dreaming a primary symptom. However, PTSD is difficult to treat and understand and resources have been committed primarily to short-term symptom suppression.[14] The resources committed to studying the science of human dreaming are miniscule, especially when compared with the resources committed to AI, neural net, and zombie systems.

But still we dream. After every night, upon awakening, many of us will remember our dreams. These dreams are more impactful, complex, and more complete than any form of equivalent cognition that can be accomplished by a machine. We understand these dreams poorly, yet we use them constantly. We use these different and alternative states of consciousness to process the complex emotions and stress of our everyday lives. We use our dreams to develop alternative approaches to what are seemingly insoluble problems when addressed in waking focus. Dreams help us to response flexibly to our species' rapidly changing external environment. Individually, we accept our capacity to dream. We apply and use the experience in any way we can. But socially and scientifically, we approach dreams differently, often suppressing the possibility that our dreams have any importance. We attempt to escape from the feedback our dreams provide. We wander outside Plato's cave into the waking world, dazed, and blinded in the light.

In the light of day, most of us interact with parametrically programmed computers on a routine basis. We attempt to force our sometimes illogical, shades-of-gray reasoning into interaction with a digital yes/no interface constructed with a logical theory of mind. More often than not that interaction is frustrating. In computer-interactive jobs and social interactions, we are routinely confronted with confusion and frustration, which we express in anthropomorphic anger towards our creations. Uncomfortable with the constraints of black-and-white logic, we become more extreme in our expressions and beliefs. Rational logic, structured with a theory of mind, can become viewed as inhuman, even possibly irrelevant to our commonsense human existence.

If our interacting machines could express a psychodynamic of emotions, it is likely that they would express frustration as well. That frustration might look like dysfunction—the robot falling over as it attempts to climb stairs, or the personal computer locked into the spinning wheel of death (SWOD) after an overload of contradictory instructions. In frustration-based anger, the machine tries to force the human into developing a logical theory of mind: in requiring yes or no answers; in adhering to set protocols; and in requiring coherent responses. This is often the typical human—computer interaction of today.

We may be unsure of the importance of dreaming, and unclear as to how to use the experience, but we are beginning to understand that dreams intrinsically affect our behavior. Our dreams personify the irrationality, uniqueness, emotional difficulty, and creativity of the human experience. If we are to interact with AI in our sometimes-illogical world, we will need to extend the capacity for commonsense functioning to our artificial creations. Otherwise, we will continue to be forced to adapt our logic to meet the parametric criteria of our machines. Instead we can attempt to teach our machines to interact with us in the same fashion in which we interact with each other.

There is a very real, potential future scenario in which we join our machines in entering alternative worlds of dream. Within this dyad, we may become immensely more knowledgeable, powerful, and insightful. For better and worse, our portion of the cognitive cyborg will still be human, still confused, still unsure of the experience of reality, and using the counterpoint unreality of dream primarily to make our waking experience more real. We sometimes dismiss dreams, possessed with no more perspective and intelligence than before our connection to the interface. Perhaps when we are able to create our super-intelligent doppelganger, our anthropomorphic dream machine, we will begin to understand the remarkable nature of dreams.

## Notes

1. Plato (380 BC). The cave: The third stage. The genuine liberation of man to the primordial light-part 1, *The Republic*. Rouse, W. H. D. (Ed.). (2008). *The Republic Book VII* (pp. 365–401). New York: Penguin Group Inc.
2. Canales, J. (2015). *The physicist and the philosopher Einstein, Bergson, and the debate that changed Our understanding of time*. Princeton, NJ: Princeton University Press.
3. King, M. L. (August 28, 1963). *I had a dream speech*. National Archives and Records Administration.
4. Vann, B., & Alperstein, N. (2000). Dream sharing as social interaction. *Dreaming, 10*, 111. The Sociology of Dreams is an aspect of the field in serious need of further study.
5. Pagel, J. F., & Vann, B. (1992). The effects of dreaming on awake behavior. *Dreaming, 2*(4), 229–223; Pagel, J. F., & Vann, B. (1993). Cross-cultural dream use in Hawaii. *Hawaii Medical Journal, 52*(2), 44–45.
6. Pagel, J. F., & Scrima, L. (2010). Psychoanalysis and narcolepsy. In M. Goswami, S. R. Pandi-Perumal, & M. Thorpy (Eds.), *Narcolepsy: A clinical guide* (pp. 129–134). New York: Springer/Humana Press.
7. Humphrey, N. (1998). Cave art, autism, and the evolution of the human mind. *Cambridge Archeological Journal, 8*, 165–191.
8. Pagel, J. F. (2014). *Dream science: Exploring the forms of consciousness*. Oxford: Academic Press (Elsevier).
9. Buckley, K. (2009). *Dreaming and the world's religions*. New York: New York University Press.
10. Nietzsche, F. (1976). On truth and lies in a nonmoral sense (W. Kaufmann's, Trans.). In *The portable Nietzsche*. New York: Viking Press (Original work published 1873).
11. Rothblatt, M. (2014). *Virtually human: The promise and peril of digital immorality*. New York: St. Martin's Press.
12. Stickgold, R., Malia, A., Maguire, D., Roddenberry, D., & O'Connor, M. (2000). Replaying the game: Hypnagogic images in normals and amnesics. *Science, 290*, 350.
13. Markham, H., Muller, E., Ramasuany, S., Reimann, M., Abdellah, M., Sanchez, C., et al. (2015). Reconstruction and simulation of neocortical microcircuitry. *Cell, 163*, 456–492.
14. Pagel, J. F. (2015). Treating nightmares: Sleep medicine and posttraumatic stress disorder. *Journal of Clinical Sleep Medicine, 11*(1), 9–10. In our modern world, there are very few willing to address the personal and social cost of PTSD, or the reality of a lack of treatment modalities that produce cures and/or long-term improvement.

# INDEX

*Note*: Page numbers followed by "*f*" and "*t*" refer to figures and tables, respectively.

Printed and bound by CPI Group (UK) Ltd, Croydon, CR0 4YY
08/06/2025
01896872-0001